FIRST AID

FOR THE®
PSYCHIATRY CLERKSHIP

SECOND EDITION

Series Editors:

LATHA G. STEAD, MD
Assistant Professor of Emergency Medicine
Mayo Clinic College of Medicine
Rochester, Minnesota

MATTHEW S. KAUFMAN, MD
Fellow Hematology
Long Island Jewish Medical Center
Albert Einstein College of Medicine
New Hyde Park, New York

S. MATTHEW STEAD, MD, PhD
Fellow in Pediatric Neurology
Mayo Graduate School of Medicine
Rochester, Minnesota

Faculty Advisor:

GABRIELLE J. MELIN, MS, MD
Instructor
Department of Psychiatry and Psychology
Director, Adult Psychiatry
Emergency Department Services
Mayo Clinic College of Medicine
Rochester, Minnesota

McGraw-Hill

MEDICAL PUBLISHING DIVISION

New York / Chicago / San Francisco / Lisbon / London / Madrid / Mexico City
Milan / New Delhi / San Juan / Seoul / Singapore / Sydney / Toronto

First Aid for the® Psychiatry Clerkship, Second Edition

6 7 8 9 0   QPD/QPD   0 9 8 7 6

ISBN 0-07-144872-1

Notice

Medicine is an ever-changing science. As new research and clinical experience broaden our knowledge, changes in treatment and drug therapy are required. The authors and the publisher of this work have checked with sources believed to be reliable in their efforts to provide information that is complete and generally in accord with the standards accepted at the time of publication. However, in view of the possibility of human error or changes in medical sciences, neither the authors nor the publisher nor any other party who has been involved in the preparation or publication of this work warrants that the information contained herein is in every respect accurate or complete, and they disclaim all responsibility for any errors or omissions or for the results obtained from use of the information contained in this work. Readers are encouraged to confirm the information contained herein with other sources. For example and in particular, readers are advised to check the product information sheet included in the package of each drug they plan to administer to be certain that the information contained in this work is accurate and that changes have not been made in the recommended dose or in the contraindications for administration. This recommendation is of particular importance in connection with new or infrequently used drugs.

This book was set in Goudy by Rainbow Graphics.
The editor was Catherine A. Johnson.
The production supervisor was Catherine Saggese.
Project management was provided by Rainbow Graphics.
The index was prepared by Oneida Indexing.
Quebecor World Dubuque was the printer and binder.

This book is printed on acid-free paper.

Library of Congress Cataloging-in-Publication Data

Stead, Latha G.
    First aid for the psychiatry clerkship : a student-to-student guide / Latha G. Stead, S. Matthew Stead, Matthew S. Kaufman ; faculty advisor, Gabrielle J. Melin.— 2nd ed.
        p. cm.
    ISBN 0-07-144872-1
        1. Psychiatry—Outlines, syllabi, etc. 2. Clinical clerkship—Outlines, syllabi, etc. I. Stead, S. Matthew. II. Kaufman, Matthew S. III. Title.

RC480.5.S665 2005
616.89'0071'1—dc22
                                                            2004061000

CONTENTS

INTRODUCTION

This clinical study aid was designed in the tradition of the *First Aid* series of books. It is formatted in the same way as the other books in the series; however, a stronger clinical emphasis was placed on its content in relation to psychiatry. You will find that rather than simply preparing you for success on the clerkship exam, this resource will help guide you in the clinical diagnosis and treatment of many problems seen by psychiatrists.

Each of the chapters in this book contains the major topics central to the practice of psychiatry and has been specifically designed for the medical student learning level. It contains information that psychiatry clerks are expected to learn and will ultimately be responsible for on their shelf exams.

The content of the text is organized in the format similar to other texts in the *First Aid* series. Topics are listed by bold headings, and the "meat" of the topics provides essential information. The outside margins contain mnemonics, diagrams, exam and ward tips, summary or warning statements, and other memory aids. Exam tips are marked by the icon 🗝 , tips for the wards by the icon ⚕, and clinical scenarios by the 🧍 icon.

REVIEWERS

STUDENT REVIEWERS:

EDIZA M. GIRALDEZ

Universidad Iberoamericana
Santo Domingo, Dominican Republic

KRISHNA C. VEDULA

University of Minnesota–Minneapolis
Class of 2006

RESIDENT REVIEWER:

VINAY MEHTA, MD

Senior Resident
Internal Medicine
Mayo Clinic
Rochester, Minnesota

ACKNOWLEDGMENTS

We would like to thank the following faculty for their help in reviewing the manuscript for the previous edition:

DANIEL D. COWELL, MD

Chairman
Department of Psychiatry and Behavioral Medicine
Marshall University School of Medicine
Huntington, West Virginia

DEBRA KLAMEN, MD, MPHE

Associate Professor of Psychiatry
Assistant Dean for Preclerkship Curriculum in Psychiatry
Director of Undergraduate Medical Education
University of Illinois at Chicago
Chicago, Illinois

How to Succeed in the Psychiatry Clerkship

The psychiatry clerkship can be very exciting. Depending on the type of ward or facility, you may see behavior and psychiatric profiles that are profoundly interesting as well as disturbing. A key to doing well in this clerkship is finding the balance between drawing a firm boundary of professionalism with your patients and creating a relationship of trust and comfort. After all, your patients need to share their innermost thoughts with you.

Why Spend Time on Psychiatry?

For most of you reading this book, your medical school psychiatry clerkship will encompass the entirety of your formal training in psychiatry during your career in medicine. You will see things during this rotation usually kept from the mainstream of society and medical wards. This exposure will expand your understanding of the spectrum of human cognition and behavior. Your awareness of the characteristics of mental dysfunction in psychiatric patients will serve you well in recognizing more subtle psychiatric symptoms that develop in your future patients.

The degree to which anxiety and mood disorders contribute to some patient's medical presentation cannot be overstated. In some cases there is no underlying medical problem whatsoever. Recognizing the psychiatric features of a patient's complaints can defer significant unnecessary medical workup. Furthermore, true medical illness imposes significant psychological stress, often revealing a previously subclinical psychiatric condition. Medical conditions alone and the incessant disturbances of hospitalization can stress normal cognitive function beyond its adaptive reserve, resulting in transient psychiatric symptoms.

Psychotropic medications are common in the general population. Many of these drugs have significant potential medical side effects and drug interactions. You will become familiar with these during your clerkship and will encounter them in practice regardless of your field of medicine.

Many of your patients, despite true medical illness, will benefit more from your "bedside manner" than from your prescriptions. The time you spend in this clerkship will enhance your ability to discern which of your patients require this extra attention. Providing it is the right thing for the patient and, in the long run, will require less of your energy.

And finally, it may as well be said, that generally speaking it is relatively easy to do well in this clerkship if one puts a little time into it.

▶ HOW TO BEHAVE ON THE WARDS

Respect the Patients

If you are in a city hospital and working in an inpatient ward, you will meet some people with severe mental illness. Sometimes you may want to laugh, and other times you may want to get away from them. Whatever your reaction, maintain professionalism and show the patients respect. This rule should extend to your discussions with residents and attendings; do not burst into laughter in conference, for example, while describing a patient's tendency to talk to his penis. This can be very challenging.

Respect the Field of Psychiatry

One thing a psychiatry attending hates most is a medical student who does not take the rotation seriously. Saying things like "This isn't real medicine" or "I like more scientific stuff" may drive a psychiatrist into a rage that results in a deadly evaluation. Regardless of your feelings, keep such thoughts to yourself.

Maintain Boundaries with Your Patients

It is your job to show compassion, patience, and understanding to your patients. Some might decide that you are the best doctor in the world and the only one who they will talk to. They will demand to talk to you when something does not go their way. This is a trap. Do not play the good guy when the attending decides to postpone the discharge date. True, you have to be caring, but you also have to show a unified front and make it clear that you are part of the treatment team and support the decision.

Dress in a Professional Manner

Even if the resident wears scrubs and the attending wears stiletto heels, you must dress in a professional, conservative manner. Wear a *short* white coat over your clothes unless discouraged (as in pediatrics).

Men should wear long pants, with cuffs covering the ankle; a long collared shirt; and a tie. No jeans, no sneakers, no short-sleeved shirts.

Women should wear long pants or knee-length skirt and a blouse or dressy sweater. No jeans, no sneakers, no heels greater than 1½ inches, no open-toed shoes.

Both men and women may wear scrubs occasionally, during overnight call for example. Do not make this your uniform.

Act in a Pleasant Manner

It can be stressful to be around psychiatric patients. Smooth out your experience by being nice to be around. Smile a lot and learn everyone's name. If you do not understand or disagree with a treatment plan or diagnosis, do not "challenge." Instead, say "I'm sorry, I don't quite understand, could you please explain. . . ." Be empathetic toward patients.

Be Aware of the Hierarchy

The way in which this will affect you will vary from hospital to hospital and team to team, but it is always present to some degree. In general, address your questions regarding ward functioning to interns or residents. Address your medical questions to attendings; make an effort to be somewhat informed on your subject prior to asking attendings medical questions.

Address Patients and Staff in a Respectful Way

Address patients as Sir, Ma'am, or Mr., Mrs., or Miss. Try not to address patients as "honey," "sweetie," and the like. Although you may feel these names are friendly, patients will think you have forgotten their name, that you are being inappropriately familiar, or both. Address all physicians as "doctor," unless told otherwise.

Take Responsibility for Your Patients

Know everything there is to know about your patients: their history, test results, details about their psychiatric and medical problems, and prognosis. Keep your intern or resident informed of new developments that they might not be aware of, and ask them for any updates you might not be aware of. Assist the team in developing a plan; speak to consultants and family. Never deliver bad news to patients or family members without the assistance of your supervising resident or attending.

Respect Patients' Rights

1. All patients have the right to have their personal medical information kept private. This means do not discuss the patient's information with family members without that patient's consent, and do not discuss any patient in hallways, elevators, or cafeterias.
2. All patients have the right to refuse treatment. This means they can refuse treatment by a specific individual (you, the medical student), or of a specific type (no electroconvulsive therapy). Patients can even refuse life-saving treatment. The only exceptions to this rule are if the patient is deemed to not have the capacity to make decisions or understand situations, in which case a health care proxy should be sought, or if the patient is suicidal or homicidal.
3. All patients should be informed of the right to seek advanced directives on admission. Often, this is done by the admissions staff, in a booklet. If your patient is chronically ill or has a life-threatening illness, address the subject of advanced directives with the assistance of your attending.

Volunteer

Be self-propelled, self-motivated. Volunteer to help with a procedure or a difficult task. Volunteer to give a 20-minute talk on a topic of your choice. Volunteer to take additional patients. Volunteer to stay late.

Be a Team Player

Help other medical students with their tasks; teach them information you have learned. Support your supervising intern or resident whenever possible. Never steal the spotlight or make a fellow medical student look bad.

Keep Patient Information Handy

Use a clipboard, notebook, or index cards to keep patient information, including a miniature history and physical, and lab and test results, at hand.

Present Patient Information in an Organized Manner

Here is a template for the "bullet" presentation:

"This is a [age]-year-old [gender] with a history of [major history such as bipolar disorder] who presented on [date] with [major symptoms, such as auditory hallucinations] and was found to have [working diagnosis]. [Tests done] showed [results]. Yesterday, the patient [state important changes, new plan, new tests, new medications]. This morning the patient feels [state the patient's words], and the psychiatric and physical exams are significant for [state major findings]. Plan is [state plan].

The newly admitted patient generally deserves a longer presentation following the complete history and physical format.

Some patients have extensive histories. The whole history should be present in the admission note, but in ward presentation, it is often too much to absorb. In these cases, it will be very much appreciated by your team if you can generate a **good summary** that maintains an accurate picture of the patient. This usually takes some thought, but it's worth it.

▶ HOW TO PREPARE FOR THE CLERKSHIP (SHELF) EXAM

If you have read about your core psychiatric illnesses and core symptoms, you will know a great deal about psychiatry. To study for the clerkship or shelf exam, we recommend:

2 or 3 weeks before exam: Read this entire review book, taking notes.
10 days before exam: Read the notes you took during the rotation on your core content list and the corresponding review book sections.
5 days before exam: Read this entire review book, concentrating on lists and mnemonics.
2 days before exam: Exercise, eat well, skim the book, and go to bed early.
1 day before exam: Exercise, eat well, review your notes and the mnemonics, and go to bed on time. Do not have any caffeine after 2 P.M.

Other helpful studying strategies include:

Study with Friends

Group studying can be very helpful. Other people may point out areas that you have not studied enough and may help you focus on the goal. If you tend to get distracted by other people in the room, limit this to less than half of your study time.

Study in a Bright Room

Find the room in your house or in your library that has the best, brightest light. This will help prevent you from falling asleep. If you don't have a bright light, get a halogen desk lamp or a light that stimulates sunlight (not a tanning lamp).

Eat Light, Balanced Meals

Make sure your meals are balanced, with lean protein, fruits and vegetables, and fiber. A high-sugar, high-carbohydrate meal will give you an initial burst of energy for 1 to 2 hours, but then you'll drop.

Take Practice Exams

The point of practice exams is not so much the content that is contained in the questions, but the training of sitting still for 3 hours and trying to pick the best answer for each and every question.

SECTION II

High-Yield Facts

Examination and Diagnosis

Interviewing

MAKING THE PATIENT COMFORTABLE

The initial interview is of utmost importance to the psychiatrist. Here, he or she has the opportunity to gather vital information by maintaining a relaxed and comfortable dialogue. During the first meeting, the psychiatrist must establish a meaningful rapport with the patient. This requires that questions be asked in a quiet, comfortable setting so that the patient is at ease. The patient should feel that the psychiatrist is interested, nonjudgmental, and compassionate. Establishing trust in this manner will enable a more productive and effective interview, in turn facilitating an accurate diagnosis and treatment plan.

Taking the History

The psychiatric history follows a similar format as the history for other types of patients. It should include the following:
- Identifying data
- Chief complaint (in the patient's own words, no matter how odd sounding)
- History of present illness
- Past psychiatric history
- Past medical history
- Medications
- Allergies
- Family history
- Social history (occupation, education, living situation, substance abuse, etc.)
- Mental status exam

WHAT SHOULD THE HISTORY OF PRESENT ILLNESS INCLUDE?

- Information about current episode:
  - Why the patient came to the doctor
  - Description of current episode
  - Events leading up to current moment (precipitating events)
  - How work and relationships have been affected

- The patient's support system (who the patient lives with, distance and level of contact with friends and relatives)
- Relationship between physical and psychological symptoms
- Vegetative symptoms (i.e., insomnia, loss of appetite, problems with concentration)
- Psychotic symptoms (i.e., auditory and visual hallucinations)
- Information about past episodes:
- Chronological account of past psychiatric problems/episodes
- Establishing a baseline of mental health:
- Patient's functioning when "well"
- Developmental history—physical and intellectual ability at various stages of life (outpatient setting only)
- Life values, goals (outpatient setting)
- Evidence of secondary gain

Mental Status Examination

This is analogous to performing a physical exam in internal medicine. It is the nuts and bolts of the psychiatric exam. The mental status exam assesses the following:

- Appearance/Behavior
- Mood/Affect
- Speech
- Perception
- Thought process/Thought content
- Sensorium/Cognition
- Insight/Judgment
- Suicidal/Homicidal ideation

The mental status exam tells only about the mental status at that moment; it can change every hour or every day, etc.

Appearance

- *Physical appearance*—clothing, hygiene, posture, grooming
- *Behavior*—mannerisms, tics, eye contact
- *Attitude*—cooperative, hostile, guarded, seductive, apathetic

Speech

- *Rate*—slow, average, rapid, or pressured (*Pressured* speech is continuous, fast, and uninterruptible.)
- *Volume*—soft, average, or loud
- *Articulation*—well articulated versus lisp, stutter, mumbling
- *Tone*—angry versus pleading, etc.

Mood

Mood is the emotion that the patient tells you he feels or is conveyed nonverbally.

Affect

Affect is an assessment of how the patient's mood appears to the examiner, including the amount and range of emotional expression. It is described with the following dimensions:

To assess mood, just ask, "How are you feeling today?" It is also helpful to have patients rate their stated mood on a scale of 1 to 10.

- *Quality* describes the depth and range of the feelings shown. Parameters: Flat (none)—blunted (shallow)—constricted (limited)—full (average)—intense (more than normal)
- *Motility* describes how quickly a person appears to shift emotional states. Parameters: Sluggish—supple—labile
- *Appropriateness to content* describes whether the affect is congruent with the subject of conversation. Parameters: Appropriate—not appropriate

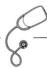

Assess the quality, motility, and appropriateness in describing the affect: "Patient's affect was constricted, sluggish, and inappropriate to content. . . ."

THOUGHT PROCESS

This is the patient's form of thinking—how he or she uses language and puts ideas together. It describes whether the patient's thoughts are logical, meaningful, and goal-directed. It does not comment on *what* the patient thinks, only *how* the patient expresses his or her thoughts.

Examples of disorders:

Loosening of associations—no logical connection from one thought to another

Flight of ideas—a fast stream of very tangential thoughts.

Neologisms—made-up words

Word salad—incoherent collection of words

Clang associations—word connections due to phonetics rather than actual meaning. "My car is red. I've been in bed. It hurts my head."

Thought blocking—abrupt cessation of communication before the idea is finished

Tangentiality—point of conversation never reached due to lack of goal-directed associations between ideas

Circumstantiality—point of conversation is reached after circuitous path

A patient who remains expressionless and monotone even when discussing extremely sad or happy moments in his life has a *flat* affect.

THOUGHT CONTENT

This describes the types of ideas expressed by the patient.

Examples of disorders:

Poverty of thought versus overabundance—too few versus too many ideas expressed

Delusions—fixed, false beliefs that are not shared by the person's culture and cannot be changed by reasoning

Suicidal and homicidal thoughts—Ask if the patient feels like harming him/herself or others. Identify if the plan is well formulated. Ask if the patient has intent (i.e., if released right now, would he go and kill himself or harm others?).

Phobias—persistent, irrational fears

Obsessions—repetitive, intrusive thoughts

Compulsions—repetitive behaviors (usually linked with obsessive thoughts)

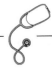

A patient who is laughing one second and crying the next has a *labile* affect.

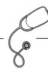

A patient who giggles while telling you that he set his house on fire and is facing criminal charges has an *inappropriate* affect.

PERCEPTION

- *Hallucinations*—sensory experiences not based in reality (visual, auditory, tactile, gustatory, olfactory)
- *Illusions*—inaccurate perception of existing sensory stimuli (Example of *illusion*: Wall appears as if it's moving)

SENSORIUM AND COGNITION

Sensorium and cognition are assessed in the following ways:

- **Consciousness**—patient's level of awareness; possible range includes: Alert—drowsy—lethargic—stuporous—coma
- **Orientation**—to person, place, and time
- **Calculation**—ability to add/subtract
- **Memory**—
  - Immediate—can repeat several digits or recall three words 5 minutes later
  - Recent—events within past few days
  - Recent past—events within past few months
  - Remote—events from childhood
- **Fund of knowledge**—level of knowledge in the context of the patient's culture and education (Who is the president? Who was Picasso?)
- **Attention/Concentration**—ability to subtract serial 7s from 100 or to spell "world" backwards
- **Reading/Writing**—simple sentences (must make sure the patient is literate first!)
- **Abstract concepts**—ability to explain similarities between objects and understand the meaning of simple proverbs

INSIGHT

This is the patient's level of awareness and understanding of his or her problem. Problems with insight include complete denial of illness or blaming it on something else.

JUDGMENT

This is the patient's ability to understand the outcome of his or her actions and use this awareness in decision making. You can ask, "What would you do if you smelled smoke in a crowded theater?"

Mini Mental State Examination (MMSE)

The MMSE is a simple, brief test used to assess gross cognitive functioning. See Cognitive Disorders chapter for detailed description. The areas tested include:

- Orientation (to person, place, and time)
- Memory (short term)
- Concentration and attention (serial 7s, spell "world" backwards)
- Language (naming, repetition, comprehension)
- Reading and writing
- Visuospatial ability (copy of design)

▶ **INTERVIEWING SKILLS**

General Approaches to Types of Patients

VIOLENT PATIENT

One should avoid being alone with a potentially violent patient. To assess violence or homicidality, one can simply ask, "Do you feel like you want to hurt someone or that you might hurt someone?" If the patient expresses imminent threats against friends, family, or others, the doctor should notify potential victims and/or protection agencies when appropriate (Tarasoff rule).

DELUSIONAL PATIENT

Although the psychiatrist should not directly challenge a delusion or insist that it is untrue, he should not imply he believes it either. He should simply acknowledge that he understands the *patient* believes the delusion is true.

DEPRESSED PATIENT

A depressed patient may be skeptical that he or she can be helped. It is important to offer reassurance that he or she can improve with appropriate therapy. Inquiring about suicidal thoughts is crucial; a feeling of hopelessness, substance use, and/or a history of prior suicide attempts reveal an increased risk for suicide. If the patient is planning or contemplating suicide, he or she must be hospitalized or otherwise protected.

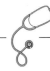

In assessing suicidality, do not simply ask, "Do you want to hurt yourself?" because this does not directly address suicidality (he may plan on dying in a painless way). Ask directly about killing self or suicide. If contemplating suicide, ask the patient if he has a plan of how to do it and if he has intent; a detailed plan, intent, and the means to accomplish it suggest a serious threat.

▶ DIAGNOSIS AND CLASSIFICATION

Diagnosis as per DSM-IV-TR Multiaxial Classification Scheme

The American Psychiatric Association uses a multiaxial classification system for diagnoses. Criteria and codes for each diagnosis are outlined in their *Diagnostic and Statistical Manual of Mental Disorders*, 4th edition, text revision (DSM-IV-TR).

Axis I: All diagnoses of mental illness (including substance abuse and developmental disorders), not including personality disorders and mental retardation

Axis II: Personality disorders and mental retardation

Axis III: General medical conditions

Axis IV: Psychosocial and environmental problems (e.g., homelessness, divorce, etc.)

Axis V: The Global Assessment of Function (GAF), which rates overall level of daily functioning (social, occupational, and psychological) on a scale of 0 to 100. (See table on next page.) Rate current GAF vs. high GAF during the past year.

▶ DIAGNOSTIC TESTING

Intelligence Tests

Aspects of intelligence include memory, logical reasoning, ability to assimilate factual knowledge, understanding of abstract concepts, etc.

INTELLIGENCE QUOTIENT (IQ)

IQ is a test of intelligence with a mean of 100 and a standard deviation of 100. These scores are adjusted for age and sometimes gender. An IQ of 100 signifies that mental age equals chronological age and corresponds to the 50th percentile in intellectual ability for the general population.

Global Assessment of Function (GAF) Scale

	1–10	11–20	21–30	31–40	41–50	51–60	61–70	71–80	81–90	91–100
Symptoms	Persistent danger of severely hurting self or others. *Recurrent violence.*	Gross impairment in communication. *Largely incoherent or mute.*	Behavior is considerably influenced by delusions or hallucinations.	Some impairment in reality testing or communication. *Speech is at times illogical, obscure, or irrelevant.*	Serious symptoms. *Suicidal ideation, severe obsessional rituals, frequent shoplifting.*	Moderate symptoms. *Flat affect and circumstantial speech, occasional panic attacks.*	Some mild symptoms. *Depressed mood, mild insomnia.*	If symptoms are present, they are transient and expectable reactions to psychosocial stressors. *Difficulty concentrating after family argument.*	Absent or minimal symptoms. *Mild anxiety before an exam.* *Generally satisfied with life.* *No more than everyday problems or concerns.* *Occasional argument with family members.*	No symptoms
Functioning	Serious suicidal act with clear expectation of death.	Some danger of hurting self or others. *Suicide attempts without clear expectation of death, frequently violent, manic excitement.*	Serious impairment in communication or judgment. *Sometimes incoherent, acts grossly inappropriately, suicidal preoccupation.*	Major impairment in several areas, such as work or school, family relations, judgment, thinking, or mood. *Depressed man avoids friends, neglects family, and is unable to work. Child frequently beats up younger children, is defiant at home and is failing in school.*	Any serious impairment in social, occupational, or school functioning. *No friends, unable to keep a job.*	Moderate difficulty in social, occupational, or school functioning. *Few friends, conflicts with co-workers.*	Some difficulty in social, occupational, or school functioning. *Occasional truancy, or theft within the household, but generally functioning pretty well, has some meaningful interpersonal relationships.*	No more than slight impairment in social, occupational, or school functioning. *Temporarily falling behind in school work.*	Good functioning in all areas, interested and involved in a wide range of activities, socially effective.	Superior functioning in a wide range of activities. *Life's problems never seem to get out of hand.*
	Persistent inability to maintain minimal personal hygiene.	Occasionally fails to maintain minimal personal hygiene *Smears feces.*	Inability to function in almost all areas. *Stays in bed all day, no job, home, or friends.*							Sought out by others because of his or her many positive qualities.

14

Intelligence tests assess cognitive function by evaluating comprehension, fund of knowledge, math skills, vocabulary, picture assembly, and other verbal and performance skills. Two common tests are:

Wechsler Adult Intelligence Scale (WAIS)
- Most common test for ages 16 to 75
- Assesses overall intellectual functioning
- Two parts: Verbal and visual-spatial

Stanford–Binet Test
- Tests intellectual ability in patients ages 2 to 18

IQ Chart
Very superior: > 130
Superior: 120–129
High average: 110–119
Average: 90–109
Low average: 80–89
Borderline: 70–79
Mild mental retardation: 50–70
Moderate mental retardation: 35–49
Severe mental retardation: 25–34
Profound mental retardation: < 25

Objective Personality Assessment Tests

These tests are questions with standardized-answer format that can be objectively scored. The following is an example:

Minnesota Multiphasic Personality Inventory (MMPI-2)
- Tests personality for different pathologies and behavioral patterns
- Most commonly used

Projective (Personality) Assessment Tests

Projective tests have no structured-response format. The tests often ask for interpretation of ambiguous stimuli. Examples are:

Thematic Apperception Test (TAT)
- Test-taker creates stories based on pictures of people in various situations.
- Used to evaluate motivations behind behaviors

Rorschach Test
- Interpretation of ink blots
- Used to identify thought disorders and defense mechanisms

Psychotic Disorders

Psychosis is a break from reality involving delusions, perceptual disturbances, and/or disordered thinking. Schizophrenia and substance-induced psychosis are examples of commonly diagnosed psychotic disorders.

Includes disorders of thought *content* and thought *process* (see chapter on Examination and Diagnosis for further clarification):

- Disorders of thought *content* reflect the patient's beliefs, ideas, and interpretations of his or her surroundings. (*Examples:* Paranoid delusions, ideas of reference, and loss of ego boundaries)
- Disorders of thought *process* involve the manner in which the patient links ideas and words together. (*Examples:* Tangentiality, circumstantiality, loosening of associations, thought blocking, perseveration, etc.)

Fixed, false beliefs that cannot be altered by rational arguments and cannot be accounted for by the cultural background of the individual

Types

- **Paranoid delusion**—irrational belief that one is being persecuted ("The CIA is after me and taps my phone.")
- **Ideas of reference**—belief that some event is uniquely related to the individual ("Jesus is speaking to me through TV characters.")
- **Thought broadcasting**—belief that one's thoughts can be heard by others
- **Delusions of grandeur**—belief that one has special powers beyond those of a normal person ("I am the all-powerful son of God and I shall bring down my wrath on you if I cannot have a smoke.")
- **Delusions of guilt**—false belief that one is guilty or responsible for something ("I caused the flood in Mozambique.")

Clinically, one can quickly tell that a person is psychotic by the presence of any one of the following:
- Perceptual disturbances (hallucinations)
- Delusional thinking
- Disordered thought process

Hallucination

Sensory perception without an actual external stimulus

Types
- **Auditory** hallucination—most commonly exhibited by schizophrenic patients
- **Visual** hallucination—commonly seen with drug intoxication
- **Olfactory** hallucination—usually an aura associated with epilepsy
- **Tactile** hallucination—usually secondary to drug abuse or alcohol withdrawal

Illusion

Misinterpretation of an existing sensory stimulus (such as mistaking a shadow for a cat)

► **DIFFERENTIAL DIAGNOSIS OF PSYCHOSIS**

- Psychosis secondary to general medical condition
- Substance-induced psychotic disorder
- Delirium/Dementia
- Bipolar disorder
- Major depression with psychotic features
- Brief psychotic disorder
- Schizophrenia
- Schizophreniform disorder
- Schizoaffective disorder
- Delusional disorder

► **PSYCHOSIS SECONDARY TO GENERAL MEDICAL CONDITION**

Medical causes of psychosis include:

1. *CNS disease* (cerebrovascular disease, multiple sclerosis, neoplasm, Parkinson's disease, Huntington's chorea, temporal lobe epilepsy, encephalitis, prion disease)
2. *Endocrinopathies* (Addison's/Cushing's disease, hyper/hypothyroidism, hyper/hypocalcemia, hypopituitarism)
3. *Nutritional/Vitamin deficiency states* (B_{12}, folate, niacin)
4. *Other* (connective tissue disease [systemic lupus erythematosus, temporal arteritis], porphyria)

Sidebar:

HIGH-YIELD FACTS

Psychotic Disorders

Loss of ego boundaries: Unawareness of where one's mind and body end and those of others begin

Differential of Psychosis
- Psychosis secondary to general medical condition
- Substance-induced psychotic disorder
- Delirium/Dementia
- Bipolar disorder
- Major depression with psychotic features
- Brief psychotic disorder
- Schizophrenia
- Schizophreniform disorder
- Schizoaffective disorder
- Delusional disorder

Always be sure to include the importance of ruling out medical, neurological, or substance-induced conditions.

DSM-IV criteria for psychotic disorder secondary to a general medical condition include:

- Prominent hallucinations or delusions
- Symptoms do not occur only during episode of delirium
- Evidence to support medical cause from lab data, history, or physical

Causes of medication/substance-induced psychosis include antidepressants, antiparkinsonian agents, antihypertensives, antihistamines, anticonvulsants, digitalis, beta blockers, antituberculosis agents, corticosteroids, hallucinogens, amphetamines, opiates, bromide, heavy metal toxicity, and alcohol.

DSM-IV Criteria
- Prominent hallucinations or delusions
- Symptoms do not occur only during episode of delirium
- Evidence to support medication or substance-related cause from lab data, history, or physical
- Disturbance is not better accounted for by a psychotic disorder that is not substance-induced.

Schizophrenia is a psychiatric disorder characterized by a constellation of abnormalities in thinking, emotion, and behavior. There is no single symptom that is pathognomonic, and the disease can produce a wide spectrum of clinical pictures. It is usually chronic and debilitating.

Positive and Negative Symptoms

In general, the symptoms of schizophrenia are broken up into two categories:
- **Positive** symptoms—hallucinations, delusions, bizarre behavior, or thought disorder
- **Negative** symptoms—blunted affect, anhedonia, apathy, and inattentiveness. Although negative symptoms are the less dramatic of the two types, they are considered by some to be at the "core" of the disorder.

Three Phases

Symptoms of schizophrenia usually present in three phases:

1. **Prodromal**—decline in functioning that precedes the first psychotic episode. The patient may become socially withdrawn and irritable. He or she may have physical complaints and/or newfound interest in religion or the occult.
2. **Psychotic**—perceptual disturbances, delusions, and disordered thought process/content
3. **Residual**—occurs between episodes of psychosis. It is marked by flat affect, social withdrawal, and odd thinking or behavior (negative symptoms). Patients can continue to have hallucinations even with treatment.

To make the diagnosis of schizophrenia, a patient must have symptoms of the disease for at least 6 months.

A 22-year-old college student has been staying in his room most of the time and avoiding his social activities. His friends have noticed that over the past 9 months, "he has been very religious" and often talks about the meaning of life. He reveals to you that he is "Jesus" and his purpose of existence is to save the human race. *Think: Schizophrenia.*

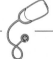

> 5 **A**s of schizophrenia
> (negative symptoms):
> 1. **A**nhedonia
> 2. **A**ffect (flat)
> 3. **A**logia (poverty of speech)
> 4. **A**volition (apathy)
> 5. **A**ttention (poor)

> **Echolalia**—repeats words or phrases
> **EchoPRAxia**—mimics behavior (**PRA**ctices behavior)

Diagnosis of Schizophrenia

DSM-IV Criteria
- *Two or more* of the following must be present for at least *1 month:*
  1. Delusions
  2. Hallucinations
  3. Disorganized speech
  4. Grossly disorganized or catatonic behavior
  5. Negative symptoms (such as flattened affect)
- Must cause significant social or occupational functional deterioration
- Duration of illness for at least 6 months (including prodromal or residual periods in which above criteria may not be met)
- Symptoms not due to medical, neurological, or substance-induced disorder

Subtypes of Schizophrenia

Patients are further subdivided into the following five subtypes:

1. **Paranoid type**—highest functioning type, older age of onset. Must meet the following criteria:
   - Preoccupation with one or more delusions or frequent auditory hallucinations
   - No predominance of disorganized speech, disorganized or catatonic behavior, or inappropriate affect
2. **Disorganized type**—poor functioning type, early onset. Must meet the following criteria:
   - Disorganized speech
   - Disorganized behavior
   - Flat or inappropriate affect
3. **Catatonic type**—rare. Must meet at least two of the following criteria:
   - Motor immobility
   - Excessive purposeless motor activity
   - Extreme negativism or mutism
   - Peculiar voluntary movements or posturing
   - **Echolalia** or **echopraxia**
4. **Undifferentiated type**—characteristic of more than one subtype or none of the subtypes
5. **Residual type**—prominent *negative* symptoms (such as flattened affect or social withdrawal) with only minimal evidence of positive symptoms (such as hallucinations or delusions)

Psychiatric Exam of Schizophrenics

The typical findings in schizophrenic patients on exam include:
- Disheveled appearance
- Flattened affect
- Disorganized thought process
- Intact memory and orientation
- Auditory hallucinations
- Paranoid delusions
- Ideas of reference (feel references are being made to them by the television or newspaper, etc.)
- Concrete understanding of similarities/proverbs
- Lack insight into their disease

Epidemiology

- Schizophrenia affects approximately 1% of people over their lifetime.
- Men and women are equally affected but have different presentations and outcomes:
  - Men tend to present around 20 years of age.
  - Women present closer to 30 years of age.
  - The course of the disease is generally more severe in men, as men tend to have more negative symptoms and are less able to function in society.
- Schizophrenia rarely presents before age 15 or after age 45.
- There is a strong genetic predisposition:
  - 50% concordance rate among monozygotic twins
  - 40% risk of inheritance if both parents have schizophrenia
  - 12% risk if one first-degree relative is affected
- There is a strong association with substance use which may be a form of self medication and depression. Postpsychotic depression occurs in 50% of patients.

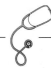

People born in winter and early spring have a higher incidence of schizophrenia for unknown reasons. (One theory involves seasonal variation in viral infections of mothers during pregnancy.)

Downward Drift

Lower socioeconomic groups have higher rates of schizophrenia. This may be due to the **downward drift hypothesis,** which postulates that people suffering from schizophrenia are unable to function well in society and hence enter lower socioeconomic groups. Many homeless people in urban areas suffer from schizophrenia.

Pathophysiology of Schizophrenia: The Dopamine Hypothesis

Though the exact cause of schizophrenia is not known, it appears to be partly related to increased dopamine activity in certain neuronal tracts. Evidence to support this hypothesis is that most antipsychotics that are successful in treating schizophrenia are dopamine receptor antagonists. In addition, cocaine and amphetamines increase dopamine activity and can lead to schizophrenic-like symptoms.

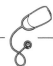

It is often impossible to differentiate an acute psychotic episode related to schizophrenia from one related to cocaine or amphetamine abuse, as these drugs excite dopaminergic pathways.

Theorized Dopamine Pathways Affected in Schizophrenia
- *Prefrontal cortical*—responsible for negative symptoms
- *Mesolimbic*—responsible for positive symptoms

Other Important Dopamine Pathways Affected by Neuroleptics
- *Tuberoinfundibular*—blocked by neuroleptics, causing hyperprolactinemia
- *Nigrostriatal*—blocked by neuroleptics, causing extrapyramidal side effects

Other Neurotransmitter Abnormalities Implicated in Schizophrenia

Elevated serotonin—some of the atypical antipsychotics (such as risperidone and clozapine) antagonize serotonin (in addition to their effects on dopamine).

Elevated norepinephrine—long-term use of antipsychotics has been shown to decrease activity of noradrenergic neurons.

Decreased gamma-aminobutyric acid (GABA)—recent data support the

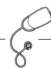

CT scans of patients with schizophrenia often show enlargement of the ventricles and diffuse cortical atrophy.

hypothesis that schizophrenic patients have a loss of GABAergic neurons in the hippocampus; this loss might indirectly activate dopaminergic and noradrenergic pathways.

PROGNOSTIC FACTORS

Schizophrenia is usually chronic and debilitating. Forty to 50% of patients remain significantly impaired after their diagnosis, while only 20 to 30% function fairly well in society with medication. Several factors are associated with a better or worse prognosis:

Associated with Better Prognosis
- Later onset
- Good social support
- Positive symptoms
- Mood symptoms
- Acute onset
- Female sex
- Few relapses
- Good premorbid functioning

Associated with Worse Prognosis
- Early onset
- Poor social support
- Negative symptoms
- Family history
- Gradual onset
- Male sex
- Many relapses
- Poor premorbid functioning (social isolation, etc.)

TREATMENT

A multimodality approach is the most effective, and therapy must be tailored to the needs of the specific patient. **Pharmacologic** treatment consists primarily of antipsychotic medications, otherwise known as neuroleptics. (For more detail, see Psychopharmacology chapter.)
- **Typical neuroleptics:** *Chlorpromazine, thioridazine, trifluoperazine, haloperidol.* These are dopamine (mostly D_2) antagonists. They are classically better at treating positive symptoms than negative. They have important side effects and sequelae such as extrapyramidal symptoms, neuroleptic malignant syndrome, and tardive dyskinesia (see below).
- **Atypical neuroleptics:** *Risperidone, clozapine, olanzapine, quetiapine, aripiprazole, ziprosidone.* These antagonize serotonin receptors ($5\text{-}HT_2$) as well as dopamine receptors. Atypical neuroleptics are classically better at treating negative symptoms than traditional neuroleptics. They have a much lower incidence of extrapyramidal side effects.
- Medications should be taken for at least 4 weeks before efficacy is determined. If the medication fails, it is appropriate to switch to another medication in a different class.

Behavioral therapy attempts to improve patients' ability to function in society. Patients are helped through a variety of methods to improve their social skills, become self-sufficient, and act appropriately in public. **Family therapy** and **group therapy** are also useful adjuncts.

Significant improvement is noted in 70% of schizophrenic patients who take antipsychotic medication.

Important Side Effects and Sequelae of Antipsychotic Medications

Side effects of antipsychotic medications include:

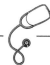

1. Extrapyramidal symptoms (especially with the use of high-potency traditional antipsychotics):
   - Dystonia (spasms) of face, neck, and tongue
   - Parkinsonism (resting tremor, rigidity, bradykinesia)
   - Akathisia (feeling of restlessness)

   Treatment: Antiparkinsonian agents (benztropine, amantadine, etc.), benzodiazepines

2. Anticholinergic symptoms (especially low-potency traditional antipsychotics and atypical antipsychotics):
   - Dry mouth, constipation, blurred vision

   Treatment: As per symptom (eyedrops, stool softeners, etc.)

3. Tardive dyskinesia (high-potency antipsychotics):
   - Darting or writhing movements of face, tongue, and head

   Treatment: Discontinue offending agent and substitute atypical neuroleptic. Benzodiazepines, beta blockers, and cholinomimetics may be used short term. The movements often persist despite withdrawal of the offending drug.

4. Neuroleptic malignant syndrome (high-potency antipsychotics):
   - Confusion, high fever, elevated blood pressure, tachycardia, "lead pipe" rigidity, sweating, and greatly elevated creatine phosphokinase (CPK) levels
   - Can be life-threatening. Is not an "allergic" reaction to a drug.

5. Weight gain, sedation, orthostatic hypotension, electrocardiogram changes, hyperprolactinemia (leading to gynecomastia, galactorrhea, amenorrhea, diminished libido, and impotence), hematologic effects (agranulocytosis may occur with *clozapine,* necessitating weekly blood draws when this medication is used), ophthalmologic conditions (*thioridazine* may cause irreversible retinal pigmentation at high doses; deposits in lens and cornea may occur with *chlorpromazine*), dermatologic conditions (such as rashes and photosensitivity), hyperlipemia, and glucose intolerance.

High-potency neuroleptics (such as haloperidol and trifluoperazine) have a higher incidence of extrapyramidal side effects than anticholinergic, while *low-potency* neuroleptics (such as chlorpromazine and thioridazine) have primarily anticholinergic side effects.

Tardive dyskinesia occurs most often in older women after at least 6 months of medication. Though 50% of patients will experience spontaneous remission, prompt discontinuation of the agent is important because the condition may become permanent.

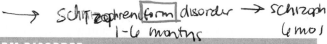

(handwritten) → Schizophreniform disorder → Schizoph 1–6 months   6 mos

> ## ► SCHIZOPHRENIFORM DISORDER

DIAGNOSIS AND DSM-IV CRITERIA

The diagnosis of schizophreniform disorder is made using the same DSM-IV criteria as schizophrenia. The only difference between the two is that in schizophreniform disorder the symptoms have lasted between 1 and 6 months, whereas in schizophrenia the symptoms must be present for more than 6 months.

PROGNOSIS

One third of patients recover completely; two thirds progress to schizoaffective disorder or schizophrenia.

TREATMENT

Hospitalization, 3- to 6-month course of antipsychotics, and supportive psychotherapy

Neuroleptic malignant syndrome is most common in men who have recently begun medication. It is considered a medical emergency, as it is associated with a 20% mortality rate. Discontinue medication immediately.

For the past 7 weeks, a 25-year-old medical student has been living in his car despite having adequate housing. He claims that the FBI has put cameras in his dorm room to monitor his every action. His friends state that lately he has been withdrawn and rarely shows up for lectures. He exhibits looseness of association, poor insight, and is concrete to proverbs. *Think: Schizophreniform disorder.*

A 33-year-old male is brought in because he tried to light his body on fire. He tearfully states that satan is trying to freeze his body. In the past winter, he never went outside for this reason and describes feeling sad to a point that he wanted to kill himself. Further questioning reveals that he had a few similar episodes over the last 10 years. When he was treated with risperidone and sertraline, his mood symptoms resolves but his delusions persisted. *Think: Schizoaffective disorder.*

SchizophreniniFORM = the FORMation of a schizophrenic, but not quite there (i.e., < 6 months).

► **SCHIZOAFFECTIVE DISORDER**

DIAGNOSIS AND DSM-IV CRITERIA

The diagnosis of schizoaffective disorder is made in patients who:

- Meet criteria for either major depressive episode, manic episode, or mixed episode (during which criteria for schizophrenia are also met)
- Have had delusions or hallucinations for 2 weeks in the absence of mood disorder symptoms (this condition is necessary to differentiate schizoaffective disorder from mood disorder with psychotic features)
- Have mood symptoms present for substantial portion of psychotic illness
- Symptoms not due to general medical condition or drugs

PROGNOSIS

Better than schizophrenia but worse than mood disorder

TREATMENT

- Hospitalization and supportive psychotherapy
- Medical therapy: Antipsychotics as needed for short-term control of psychosis; mood stabilizers, antidepressants, or electroconvulsive therapy (ECT) as needed for mania or depression

---

► **BRIEF PSYCHOTIC DISORDER**

DIAGNOSIS AND DSM-IV CRITERIA

Patient with psychotic symptoms as defined for schizophrenia; however, the symptoms last from 1 day to 1 month. Symptoms must not be due to general medical condition or drugs. This is a rare diagnosis, much less common than schizophrenia.

PROGNOSIS

Fifty to 80% recovery rate; 20 to 50% may eventually be diagnosed with schizophrenia or mood disorder.

TREATMENT

Brief hospitalization, supportive psychotherapy, course of antipsychotics for psychosis itself and/or benzodiazepines for agitation

Comparing Time Courses and Prognoses of Psychotic Disorders

Time Course
< 1 month—brief psychotic disorder
1–6 months—schizophreniform disorder
> 6 months—schizophrenia

Prognosis from Best to Worst
Mood disorder > brief psychotic disorder > schizoaffective disorder > schizophreniform disorder > schizophrenia

Delusional disorder occurs more often in older patients (after age 40), immigrants, and the hearing impaired.

DIAGNOSIS AND DSM-IV CRITERIA

To be diagnosed with delusional disorder, the following criteria must be met (see Table 3-1):
- Nonbizarre, fixed delusions for at least 1 month
- Does not meet criteria for schizophrenia
- Functioning in life not significantly impaired

Types of Delusions

Patients are further categorized based on the types of delusions they experience:
- **Erotomanic type**—delusion revolves around love (Eros is the goddess of love)
- **Grandiose type**—inflated self-worth
- **Somatic type**—physical delusions
- **Persecutory type**—delusions of being persecuted
- **Jealous type**—delusions of unfaithfulness
- **Mixed type**—more than one of the above

PROGNOSIS

50% full recovery, 20% decreased symptoms, and 30% no change

TREATMENT

Psychotherapy may be helpful. Antipsychotic medications are often ineffective, but a course of them should be tried (usually a high-potency traditional antipsychotic or one of the newer atypical antipsychotics is used).

Two weeks after the death of her 6-month-old infant, a 30-year-old female is brought into the ER because she says she hears the infant crying in the next room. She often carries a pillow in her arms and sings nursery rhymes to it. *Think: Brief psychotic disorder.*

Nonbizarre delusions: Beliefs that might occur in real life but are not currently true (such as having a disease, having an unfaithful spouse, etc.) *Bizarre* delusions: Beliefs that have no basis in reality (such as aliens living in the attic, etc.)

HIGH-YIELD FACTS

Psychotic Disorders

TABLE 3-1. Schizophrenia vs. Delusional Disorder

Schizophrenia	Delusional Disorder
■ Bizarre delusions (or nonbizarre)	■ Nonbizarre delusions (never bizarre)
■ Daily functioning significantly impaired	■ Daily functioning not significantly impaired

■ Must have two or more of the following:
  ■ Delusions
  ■ Hallucinations
  ■ Disorganized speech
  ■ Disorganized behavior
  ■ Negative symptoms
	■ Does not meet the criteria for schizophrenia as described in left column

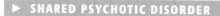

DIAGNOSIS AND DSM-IV CRITERIA

Also known as *folie à deux*, shared psychotic disorder is diagnosed when a patient develops the same delusional symptoms as someone he or she is in a close relationship with. Most people suffering from shared psychotic disorder are family members.

PROGNOSIS

Twenty to 40% will recover upon removal from the inducing person.

TREATMENT

The first step is to separate the patient from the person who is the source of shared delusions (usually a family member with an underlying psychotic disorder). Psychotherapy should be undertaken, and antipsychotic medications should be used if symptoms have not improved in 1 to 2 weeks after separation.

▶ **CULTURE-SPECIFIC PSYCHOSES**

These are psychoses seen only within certain cultures:

	Psychotic Manifestation	**Culture**
Koro	Patient believes that his penis is shrinking and will disappear, causing his death.	Asia
Amok	Sudden unprovoked outbursts of violence of which the person has no recollection. Person often commits suicide afterwards.	Malaysia, Southeast Asia
Brain fag	Headache, fatigue, and visual disturbances in male students	Africa

▶ **QUICK AND EASY DISTINGUISHING FEATURES**

- **Schizophrenia**—lifelong psychotic disorder
- **Schizophreniform**—schizophrenia for < 6 months
- **Schizoaffective**—schizophrenia + mood disorder
- **Schizotypal** (personality disorder)—paranoid, odd or magical beliefs, eccentric, lack of friends, social anxiety. Criteria for true psychosis are not met.
- **Schizoid** (personality disorder)—withdrawn, lack of enjoyment from social interactions, emotionally restricted

Mood Disorders

▶ **CONCEPTS IN MOOD DISORDERS**

A **mood** is a description of one's internal emotional state. Both external and internal stimuli can trigger moods, which may be labeled as sad, happy, angry, irritable, and so on. It is normal to have a wide range of moods and to have a sense of control over one's moods.

Patients with mood *disorders* experience an abnormal range of moods and lose some level of control over them. Distress may be caused by the severity of their moods and their resulting impairment in social and occupational functioning.

Mood disorders have also been called **affective disorders.**

Mood Disorders Versus Mood Episodes

Mood episodes are distinct periods of time in which some abnormal mood is present. Mood disorders are defined by their patterns of mood episodes.

Types of Mood Episodes

- Major depressive episode
- Manic episode
- Mixed episode
- Hypomanic episode

The Main Mood Disorders

- Major depressive disorder (MDD)
- Bipolar I disorder
- Bipolar II disorder
- Dysthymic disorder
- Cyclothymic disorder

Some may have psychotic features (delusions or hallucinations).

Major depressive episodes can be present in either major depressive disorder or bipolar I/II disorder.

Symptoms of major depression:
Sleep
Interest
Guilt

Energy

Concentration
Appetite
Psychomotor activity
Suicidal ideation

A manic episode is a *psychiatric emergency;* severely impaired judgment makes patient dangerous to self and others.

Symptoms of mania:
DIG FAST
Distractability
Insomnia
Grandiosity

Flight of ideas
Activity/agitation
Speech (pressured)
Thoughtlessness

Irritability is usually the predominant mood state in mixed episodes. Patients with mixed episodes have a poorer response to lithium. Anticonvulsants may help.

Major Depressive Episode (DSM-IV Criteria)

Must have at least five of the following symptoms (must include either number 1 or number 2) for at least a 2-week period:

1. Depressed mood
2. Anhedonia (loss of interest in pleasurable activities)
3. Change in appetite or body weight (increased or decreased)
4. Feelings of worthlessness or excessive guilt
5. Insomnia or hypersomnia
6. Diminished concentration
7. Psychomotor agitation or retardation (i.e., restlessness or slowness)
8. Fatigue or loss of energy
9. Recurrent thoughts of death or suicide

Symptoms cannot be due to substance use or medical conditions, and they must cause social or occupational impairment.

SUICIDE AND MAJOR DEPRESSIVE EPISODES

A person who has been previously hospitalized for a major depressive episode has a 15% risk of committing suicide later in life.

Manic Episode (DSM-IV Criteria)

A period of abnormally and persistently elevated, expansive, or irritable mood, lasting at least 1 week and including at least three of the following (four if mood is irritable):

1. Distractibility
2. Inflated self-esteem or grandiosity
3. Increase in goal-directed activity (socially, at work, or sexually)
4. Decreased need for sleep
5. Flight of ideas or racing thoughts
6. More talkative or *pressured speech* (rapid and uninterruptible)
7. Excessive involvement in pleasurable activities that have a high risk of negative consequences (e.g., buying sprees, sexual indiscretions)

These symptoms cannot be due to substance use or medical conditions, and they must cause social or occupational impairment. Seventy-five percent of manic patients have psychotic symptoms.

Mixed Episode

Criteria are met for both manic episode and major depressive episode. These criteria must be present nearly every day for at least 1 week. As with a manic episode, this is a psychiatric emergency.

Hypomanic Episode

A hypomanic episode is a distinct period of elevated, expansive, or irritable mood that includes at least three of the symptoms listed for the manic episode criteria (four if mood is irritable). There are significant differences between mania and hypomania (see below).

Differences Between Manic and Hypomanic Episodes

Mania
Lasts at least 7 days
Causes severe impairment in social
  or occupational functioning
May necessitate hospitalization to
  prevent harm to self or others
May have psychotic features

Hypomania
Lasts at least 4 days
No marked impairment in social or
  occupational functioning
Does not require hospitalization
No psychotic features

▶ MOOD DISORDERS

Mood disorders often have chronic courses that are marked by relapses with relatively normal functioning between episodes. Like most psychiatric diagnoses, they may be triggered by a medical condition or drug (prescribed or illicit). Always investigate medical or substance-induced causes (see below) before making a diagnosis.

Differential Diagnosis of Mood Disorders Secondary to General Medical Conditions

Medical Causes of a Depressive Episode
Cerebrovascular disease
Endocrinopathies (Cushing's
  syndrome, Addison's disease,
  hypoglycemia, hyper/
  hypothyroidism,
  hyper/hypocalcemia)
Parkinson's disease
Viral illnesses (e.g., mononucleosis)
Carcinoid syndrome
Cancer (especially lymphoma and
  pancreatic carcinoma)
Collagen vascular disease (e.g.,
  systemic lupus erythematosus)

Medical Causes of a Manic Episode

Metabolic (hyperthyroidism)
Neurological disorders (temporal
  lobe seizures, multiple sclerosis)
Neoplasms
HIV infection

Mood Disorders Secondary to Medication or Substance Use

Medication/Substance-Induced Depressive Episodes
EtOH
Antihypertensives
Barbiturates
Corticosteroids
Levodopa
Sedative–hypnotics
Anticonvulsants
Antipsychotics
Diuretics
Sulfonamides
Withdrawal from psychostimulants
  (e.g., cocaine, amphetamines)

Medication/Substance-Induced Mania
Corticosteroids
Sympathomimetics
Dopamine
Agonists
Antidepressants
Bronchodilators
Levodopa

Triad for seasonal affective disorder:
- Irritability
- Carbohydrate drawing
- Hypersomnia

► MAJOR DEPRESSIVE DISORDER (MDD)

MDD is marked by episodes of depressed mood associated with loss of interest in daily activities. Patients may be unaware of their depressed mood or may express vague, somatic complaints.

DIAGNOSIS AND DSM-IV CRITERIA

- At least one major depressive episode (see above)
- No history of manic or hypomanic episode

Seasonal affective disorder is a subtype of MDD in which major depressive episodes occur only during winter months (fewer daylight hours). Patients respond to treatment with light therapy.

EPIDEMIOLOGY

- Lifetime prevalence: 15%
- Onset at any age, but average age of onset is 40
- Twice as prevalent in women than men
- No ethnic or socioeconomic differences
- Prevalence in elderly from 25 to 50%

SLEEP PROBLEMS ASSOCIATED WITH MDD

- Multiple awakenings
- Initial and terminal insomnia (hard to fall asleep and early morning awakenings)
- Hypersomnia
- Rapid eye movement (REM) sleep shifted to earlier in night and stages 3 and 4 decreased

ETIOLOGY

The exact cause of depression is unknown, but biological, genetic, environmental, and psychosocial factors each contribute.

Abnormalities of Serotonin/Catecholamines

1. Decreased brain and cerebrospinal fluid (CSF) levels of serotonin and its main metabolite, 5-hydroxyindolacetic acid (5-HIAA), are found in depressed patients. Abnormal regulation of beta-adrenergic receptors has also been shown.
2. Drugs that increase availability of serotonin, norepinephrine, and dopamine often alleviate symptoms of depression.

Other Neuroendocrine Abnormalities

1. **High cortisol:** Hyperactivity of hypothalamic–pituitary–adrenal axis as shown by failure to suppress cortisol levels in dexamethasone suppression test.
2. **Abnormal thyroid axis:** Thyroid disorders are associated with depressive symptoms, and one third of patients with MDD who have otherwise normal thyroid hormone levels show blunted response of thyroid-stimulating hormone (TSH) to infusion of thyrotropin-releasing hormone (TRH).

These abnormalities are also associated with other psychiatric disorders; they are not specific for major depression.

Many other neurotransmitters and hormonal factors have also shown potential involvement in the pathophysiology of mood disorders, including gamma-aminobutyric acid (GABA) and endogenous opiates.

Psychosocial/Life Events

Loss of a parent before age 11 is associated with the later development of major depression. Stable family and social functioning have been shown to be good prognostic indicators in the course of major depression.

Genetic Predisposition

First-degree relatives are two to three times more likely to have MDD. Concordance rate for monozygotic twins is about 50%, and 10 to 25% for dizygotic twins.

COURSE AND PROGNOSIS

If left untreated, depressive episodes are self-limiting but usually last from 6 to 13 months. Generally, episodes occur more frequently as the disorder progresses. The risk of a subsequent major depressive episode is 50% within the first 2 years after the first episode. About 15% of patients eventually commit suicide.

Antidepressant medications significantly reduce the length and severity of symptoms. They may be used prophylactically between major depressive episodes to reduce the risk of subsequent episodes. Approximately 75% of patients are treated successfully with medical therapy.

TREATMENT

Hospitalization
- Indicated if patient is at risk for suicide, homicide, or is unable to care for self.

Pharmacotherapy

Antidepressant Medications
- Selective serotonin reuptake inhibitors (SSRIs)—safer and better tolerated than other classes of antidepressants; side effects mild but include headache, gastrointestinal disturbance, sexual dysfunction, and rebound anxiety.
- Tricyclic antidepressants (TCAs)—most lethal in overdose; side effects include sedation, weight gain, orthostatic hypotension, and anticholinergic effects. Can aggravate prolonged QTC syndrome.
- Monoamine oxidase inhibitors (MAOIs)—useful for treatment of refractory depression; risk of *hypertensive crisis* when used with sympathomimetics or ingestion of tyramine-rich foods (such as wine, beer, aged cheeses, liver, and smoked meats); risk of *serotonin syndrome* when used in combination with SSRIs. Most common side effect is orthostatic hypotension. (Tyramine is an intermediate in the conversion of tyrosine to norepinephrine.)

Adjuvant Medications
- Stimulants (such as methylphenidate) may be used in certain patients, such as the terminally ill or patients with refractory symptoms. Though action is rapid, potential for dependence limits use.

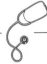

MDD may have psychotic features (delusions or hallucinations).

About two thirds of all depressed patients contemplate suicide, and 10 to 15% commit suicide.

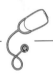

Only half of patients with MDD ever receive treatment.

All antidepressant medications are equally effective but differ in side effect profiles. Medications usually take 4 to 8 weeks to work.

Serotonin syndrome is marked by autonomic instability, hyperthermia, and seizures. Coma or death may result.

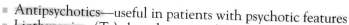

- Antipsychotics—useful in patients with psychotic features
- Liothyronine (T_3), levothyroxine (T_4), lithium, or L-tryptophan (serotonin precursor) may be added to convert nonresponders to responders.

Psychotherapy
- Behavioral therapy, cognitive therapy, supportive psychotherapy, dynamic psychotherapy, and family therapy
- May be used in conjunction with pharmacotherapy

Electroconvulsive therapy (ECT)
- Indicated if patient is unresponsive to pharmacotherapy, if patient cannot tolerate pharmacotherapy, or if rapid reduction of symptoms is desired (suicide risk, etc.)
- ECT is safe and may be used alone or in combination with pharmacotherapy.
- ECT is performed by premedication with atropine, followed by general anesthesia and administration of a muscle relaxant. A generalized seizure is then induced by passing a current of electricity across the brain (either unilateral or bilateral); the seizure lasts < 1 minute.
- Approximately eight treatments are administered over a 2- to 3-week period, but significant improvement is often noted after the first treatment.
- Retrograde amnesia is a common side effect, which usually disappears within 6 months.

Unique Types and Features of Depressive Disorders

Melancholic—40 to 60% of hospitalized patients with major depression. Characterized by anhedonia, early morning awakenings, psychomotor disturbance, excessive guilt, and anorexia. For example, you may diagnose "major depressive disorder with melancholic features."

Atypical—characterized by hypersomnia, hyperphagia, reactive mood, leaden paralysis, and hypersensitivity to interpersonal rejection

Catatonic—features include catalepsy (immobility), purposeless motor activity, extreme negativism or mutism, bizarre postures, and echolalia. May also be applied to bipolar disorder.

Psychotic—10 to 25% of hospitalized depressions. Characterized by the presence of delusions or hallucinations.

▶ **BIPOLAR I DISORDER**

Bipolar I disorder involves episodes of mania and of major depression; however, episodes of major depression are *not* required for the diagnosis. It is traditionally known as **manic depression.**

DIAGNOSIS AND DSM-IV CRITERIA

The only requirement for this diagnosis is the occurrence of one manic or mixed episode (10 to 20% of patients experience only manic episodes). Between manic episodes, there may be interspersed euthymia, major depressive episodes, dysthymia, or hypomanic episodes, but none of these are required for diagnosis.

Patients who may not be able to tolerate side effects of antidepressant medications include the elderly and pregnant women.

MAOIs are often useful in treatment of "atypical" depression.

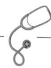

The catatonic type of major depression is usually treated with antidepressants and antipsychotics concurrently.

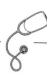

Bipolar I disorder may have **psychotic features** (delusions or hallucinations); these can occur during major depressive *or* manic episodes. Always remember to include bipolar disorder in your differential of a psychotic patient.

EPIDEMIOLOGY

- Lifetime prevalence: 1%
- Women and men equally affected
- No ethnic differences seen
- Onset usually before age 30

ETIOLOGY

Biological, environmental, psychosocial, and genetic factors are all important. First-degree relatives of patients with bipolar disorder are 8 to 18 times more likely to develop the illness. Concordance rates for monozygotic twins are approximately 75%, and rates for dizygotic twins are 5 to 25%.

COURSE AND PROGNOSIS

Untreated manic episodes generally last about 3 months. The course is usually chronic with relapses; as the disease progresses, episodes may occur more frequently. Only 7% of patients do not have a recurrence of symptoms after their first manic episode.

Bipolar disorder has a worse prognosis than MDD, as only 50 to 60% of patients treated with lithium experience significant improvement in symptoms. Lithium prophylaxis between episodes helps to decrease the risk of relapse.

TREATMENT

Pharmacotherapy
- Lithium—mood stabilizer
- Anticonvulsants (carbamazepine or valproic acid)—also mood stabilizers, especially useful for rapid cycling bipolar disorder and mixed episodes
- Olanzapine—a typical antipsychotic

Psychotherapy
- Supportive psychotherapy, family therapy, group therapy (once the acute manic episode has been controlled)

ECT
- Works well in treatment of manic episodes
- Usually requires more treatments than for depression

▶ BIPOLAR II DISORDER

Alternatively called *recurrent major depressive episodes with hypomania*

DIAGNOSIS AND DSM-IV CRITERIA

History of one or more major depressive episodes and at least one **hypomanic** episode. *Remember:* If there has been a <u>full manic episode *even in the past,*</u> then the diagnosis is *not* bipolar II disorder, but bipolar I.

A 35-year-old male is brought in by his wife because he has been taking out various loans to start a few small businesses. Over the past 2 weeks, he comes home at 3 A.M. from work and leaves at 6 A.M. and often compares his business ventures to those of Bill Gates. In the past, he has had a few episoodes in which he felt hopeless and tried to commit suicide. *Think: Bipolar disorder.*

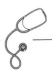

Rapid cycling is defined by the occurrence of four or more mood episodes in 1 year (major depressive, manic, mixed, etc.).

Side effects of lithium include:
- Weight gain
- Tremor
- Gastrointestinal disturbances
- Fatigue
- Arrhythmias
- Seizures
- Goiter/hypothyroidism
- Leukocytosis (benign)
- Coma
- Polyuria
- Polydipsia
- Alopecia
- Metallic taste

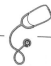

MDD tends to be episodic, while dysthymic disorder is generally persistent.

Dysthymic disorder: CHASES

- Poor **c**oncentration or difficulty making decisions
- Feelings of **h**opelessness
- Poor **a**ppetite or overeating
- In**s**omnia or hypersomnia
- Low **e**nergy or fatigue
- Low **s**elf-esteem

Dysthymic disorder (DD) = **2 Ds**

2 years of depression
2 listed criteria
Never asymptomatic for > 2 months

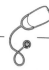

Dysthymia can never have psychotic features. If a patient has delusions or hallucinations with "depression," consider another diagnosis (e.g., major depression with psychotic features, schizoaffective, etc.).

EPIDEMIOLOGY

- Lifetime prevalence: 0.5%
- Slightly more common in women
- Onset usually before age 30
- No ethnic differences seen

ETIOLOGY

Same as bipolar I disorder (see above)

COURSE AND PROGNOSIS

Tends to be chronic, requiring long-term treatment

TREATMENT

Same as bipolar I disorder (see above)

▶ **DYSTHYMIC DISORDER**

Patients with dysthymic disorder have chronic, mild depression most of the time with no discrete episodes. They rarely need hospitalization.

DIAGNOSIS AND DSM-IV CRITERIA

1. Depressed mood for the majority of time of most days for at least 2 years (in children for at least 1 year)
2. At least two of the following:
   - Poor concentration or difficulty making decisions
   - Feelings of hopelessness
   - Poor appetite or overeating
   - Insomnia or hypersomnia
   - Low energy or fatigue
   - Low self-esteem
3. During the 2-year period:
   - The person has not been without the above symptoms for > 2 months at a time.
   - No major depressive episode

The patient must never have had a manic or hypomanic episode (this would make the diagnosis bipolar disorder or cyclothymic disorder, respectively).

Double depression: Patients with major depressive disorder with dysthymic disorder during residual periods

EPIDEMIOLOGY

- Lifetime prevalence: 6%
- Two to three times more common in women
- Onset before age 25 in 50% of patients

COURSE AND PROGNOSIS

Twenty percent of patients will develop major depression, 20% will develop bipolar disorder, and > 25% will have lifelong symptoms.

TREATMENT

- Cognitive therapy and insight-oriented psychotherapy are most effective.
- Antidepressant medications are useful when used concurrently (SSRIs, TCAs, or MAOIs).

▶ CYCLOTHYMIC DISORDER

Alternating periods of hypomania and periods with mild to moderate depressive symptoms

DIAGNOSIS AND DSM-IV CRITERIA

- Numerous periods with hypomanic symptoms and periods with depressive symptoms for at least 2 years
- The person must never have been symptom free for > 2 months during those 2 years.
- No history of major depressive episode or manic episode

EPIDEMIOLOGY

- Lifetime prevalence: < 1%
- May coexist with borderline personality disorder
- Onset usually age 15 to 25
- Occurs equally in males and females

COURSE AND PROGNOSIS

Chronic course; one third of patients eventually diagnosed with bipolar disorder

TREATMENT

Antimanic agents as used to treat bipolar disorder (see above)

▶ OTHER DISORDERS OF MOOD IN DSM-IV

- **Minor depressive disorder**—episodes of depressive symptoms that do not meet criteria for major depressive disorder; euthymic periods are also seen, unlike in dysthymic disorder.
- **Recurrent brief depressive disorder**
- **Premenstrual dysphoric disorder**
- **Mood disorder due to a general medical condition**
- **Substance-induced mood disorder**
- **Mood disorder not otherwise specified (NOS)**

A 28-year-old accountant has felt sad since her adolescence. She does not remember the last time she "did something fun." She denies any suicidal thoughts or having any episodes of hopelessness or impaired sleep pattern. *Think: Dysthymia.*

A 28-year-old graduate student says that she has her "ups and downs." Further questioning reveals that at times over the past 2 years, she has had episodes of extreme happiness in which she would party every day and felt as if "she was full of energy." She also describes being "down in the dumps" at times for no apparent reason. *Think: Cyclothymia.*

Anxiety and Adjustment Disorders

► NORMAL VERSUS PATHOLOGICAL ANXIETY

Anxiety is the subjective experience of fear and its physical manifestations. Autonomic symptoms of anxiety include palpitations, perspiration, dizziness, mydriasis, gastrointestinal disturbances, and urinary urgency and frequency. An anxious person may also experience trembling, "butterflies" in the abdomen, and tingling in the peripheral extremities. There is often a shortness of breath or choking sensation.

Anxiety is a common, normal response to a perceived threat. It is important for clinicians to be able to distinguish normal from pathological anxiety. When anxiety is pathological, it is inappropriate; there is either no real source of fear or the source is not sufficient to account for the severity of the symptoms. In people with anxiety disorders, the symptoms interfere with daily functioning and interpersonal relationships.

► ANXIETY DISORDERS

ETIOLOGY

Anxiety disorders are caused by a combination of genetic, environmental, biological, and psychosocial factors. They are associated with neurotransmitter imbalances, including increased activity of norepinephrine and decreased activity of gamma-aminobutyric acid (GABA) and serotonin.

EPIDEMIOLOGY

Anxiety disorders are very common. Women have a 30% lifetime prevalence rate, and men have a 19% lifetime prevalence rate. Anxiety disorders develop more frequently in higher socioeconomic groups.

Types of Anxiety Disorders

The primary anxiety disorders are:
- Panic disorder
- Agoraphobia
- Specific and social phobias

- Obsessive–compulsive disorder
- Posttraumatic stress disorder
- Acute stress disorder
- Generalized anxiety disorder
- Anxiety disorder secondary to general medical condition
- Substance-induced anxiety disorder

Medical Causes of Anxiety Disorders	**Medication- or Substance-Induced Anxiety Disorders**
Hyperthyroidism	Caffeine intake and withdrawal
Vitamin B_{12} deficiency	Amphetamines
Hypoxia	Alcohol and sedative withdrawal
Neurological disorders (epilepsy, brain tumors, multiple sclerosis, etc.)	Other illicit drug withdrawal
	Mercury or arsenic toxicity
Cardiovascular disease	Organophosphate or benzene toxicity
Anemia	Penicillin
Pheochromocytoma	Sulfonamides
Hypoglycemia	Sympathomimetics
	Antidepressants

Panic Attack

Panic attacks are discrete periods of heightened anxiety that classically occur in patients with panic disorder; however, they may occur in other mental disorders, especially phobic disorders and posttraumatic stress disorder.

Panic attacks often peak in several minutes and subside within 25 minutes. They rarely last > 1 hour. Attacks may be either unexpected or provoked by specific triggers. They may be described as a sudden rush of fear.

DIAGNOSIS AND DSM-IV CRITERIA

A panic attack is a discrete period of intense fear and discomfort that is accompanied by at least four of the following:
- Palpitations
- Sweating
- Shaking
- Shortness of breath
- Choking sensation
- Chest pain
- Nausea
- Light-headedness
- Depersonalization (feeling detached from oneself)
- Fear of losing control or "going crazy"
- Fear of dying
- Numbness or tingling
- Chills or hot flushes

Panic attack criteria: PANIC
Palpitations
Abdominal distress
Numbness, nausea
Intense fear of death
Choking, chills, chest pain, sweating, shaking, shortness of breath

A panic attack may be mistaken by patient for a myocardial infarction; sufferer may seek help in the emergency department (ED).

Panic Disorder

Panic disorder is characterized by the experience of panic attacks accompanied by persistent fear of having additional attacks.

DIAGNOSIS AND DSM-IV CRITERIA

1. Spontaneous recurrent panic attacks (see above) with no obvious precipitant
2. At least one of the attacks has been followed by a minimum of 1 month of the following:
   - Persistent concern about having additional attacks
   - Worry about the implications of the attack ("Am I out of control?")
   - A significant change in behavior related to the attacks (avoid situations that may provoke attacks)

Two types of diagnoses: Always specify panic disorder **with agoraphobia** or panic disorder **without agoraphobia** (see definition of agoraphobia below).

PRESENTATION

The first panic attack is usually unexpected by the patient, but it may follow a period of stress or physical exertion. In addition to physical symptoms (such as tachycardia, sweating, and shortness of breath), the patient experiences extreme fear without understanding the source or trigger of that fear. The patient may sense impending death or harm and may worry that he or she is "going crazy."

Subsequent attacks usually occur spontaneously but may be associated with specific situations. Attacks occur an average of two times per week but may range from several times per day to a few times per year. They usually last between 20 and 30 minutes, and *anticipatory anxiety* about having another attack is common between episodes.

ETIOLOGY

Biological, genetic, and psychosocial factors contribute to the development of panic disorder. Research has revealed dysregulation of the autonomic nervous system, central nervous system, and cerebral blood flow in patients with panic disorder. Increased activity of norepinephrine and decreased activity of serotonin and GABA have also been shown in these patients.

PANIC-INDUCING SUBSTANCES

Certain substances have been shown to induce panic attacks in patients with panic disorder and only infrequently trigger them in people without the disorder. For example, hyperventilation or its treatment/inhalation of carbon dioxide (CO_2) (breathing in and out of a paper bag)

In addition, caffeine and nicotine have been shown to exacerbate anxiety symptoms in patients suffering from panic disorder.

EPIDEMIOLOGY

- Lifetime prevalence: 2 to 5%
- Two to three times more common in females than males
- Strong genetic component: Four to eight times greater risk of panic disorder if first-degree relative is affected
- Onset usually from late teens to early thirties (average age 25), but may occur at any age

Consider the panic disorder diagnosis if medical workup shows no abnormalities. Studies have shown that 43% of patients presenting with chest pain and normal angiograms were diagnosed with panic disorder.

A 24-year-old female comes to the ER complaining of a pounding heart, shortness of breath, and sweating that began while she was shopping and lasted 20 minutes. She expresses that she thought she was going to die. Further questioning reveals that she has had six of these episodes in the last month and fears having another one. *Think: Panic disorder.*

The following conditions are frequently associated with both panic disorder and agoraphobia:

1. Major depression (depressive symptoms found in 40 to 80% of patients)
2. Substance dependence (found in 20 to 40% of patients)
3. Social and specific phobias
4. Obsessive–compulsive disorder

DIFFERENTIAL DIAGNOSIS

There is a vast differential diagnosis for panic disorder, including general medical conditions, substance use or withdrawal, and other mental disorders that may cause panic-like symptoms. It is important to rule out these conditions before making the diagnosis of panic disorder.

Medical: Congestive heart failure; angina; myocardial infarction; thyrotoxicosis; temporal lobe epilepsy; multiple sclerosis; pheochromocytoma; carcinoid syndrome; chronic obstructive pulmonary disease (COPD); and other cardiac, pulmonary, neurological, and endocrine abnormalities

Mental: Depressive disorders, phobic disorders, obsessive–compulsive disorder, and posttraumatic stress disorder

Drug: Amphetamine, caffeine, nicotine, cocaine, and hallucinogen intoxication; alcohol or opiate withdrawal

COURSE AND PROGNOSIS

Panic disorder has a variable course but is often chronic. Relapses are common with discontinuation of medical therapy:

- 10 to 20% of patients continue to have significant symptoms that interfere with daily functioning.
- 50% continue to have mild, infrequent symptoms.
- 30 to 40% remain free of symptoms after treatment.

TREATMENT

Pharmacological

Acute Initial Treatment of Anxiety
Benzodiazepines (only short course if necessary, as dependence may occur with long-term use); Dose should be tapered as treatment with selective serotonin reuptake inhibitors (SSRIs) is instituted.

Maintenance
SSRIs, especially paroxetine and sertraline, are the drugs of choice for long-term treatment of panic disorder. These drugs typically take 2 to 4 weeks to become effective, and higher doses are required than for depression. Clomipramine, imipramine, or other antidepressants may also be used. Treatment should continue for at least 8 to 12 months, as relapse is common after discontinuation of therapy.

Other Treatments
- Relaxation training
- Biofeedback
- Cognitive therapy
- Insight-oriented psychotherapy
- Family therapy

Always start SSRIs at low dose and increase slowly in panic disorder patients, as they are prone to develop *activation* side effects from these medications (anxiety symptoms that mimic those of panic).

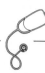

Beta blockers are *not* as effective as benzodiazepines in controlling anxiety symptoms in patients with panic disorder.

Agoraphobia

Agoraphobia is the fear of being alone in public places. It often develops secondary to panic attacks due to apprehension about having subsequent attacks in public places where escape may be difficult. It can be diagnosed alone or as panic disorder with agoraphobia; 50 to 75% of patients have coexisting panic disorder.

DIAGNOSIS AND DSM-IV CRITERIA

The following criteria must be met for diagnosis:
- Anxiety about being in places or situations from which escape might be difficult, or in which help would not be readily available in the event of a panic attack
- The situations are either avoided, endured with severe distress, or faced only with the presence of a companion.
- These symptoms cannot be better explained by another mental disorder.

TYPICAL FEARS

Characteristic situations are avoided, including being outside the home alone; being on a bridge or in a crowd; or riding in a car, bus, or train.

RELATIONSHIP BETWEEN PANIC ATTACKS AND AGORAPHOBIA

Clinical progression: A person who has a **panic attack** while shopping in a large supermarket subsequently develops a fear of entering that supermarket. As the person experiences more panic attacks in different settings, he or she develops a progressive and more general fear of public spaces **(agoraphobia).**

TREATMENT

Since agoraphobia is usually associated with panic disorder, **SSRIs** are also considered first-line treatment. Behavioral therapy may also be indicated. As coexisting panic disorder is treated, agoraphobia usually resolves. When agoraphobia is not associated with panic disorder, it is usually chronic and debilitating.

Specific and Social Phobias

A phobia is defined as an irrational fear that leads to avoidance of the feared object or situation. A *specific phobia* is a strong, exaggerated fear of a specific object or situation; a *social phobia* (also called **social anxiety disorder**) is a fear of social situations in which embarrassment can occur.

DIAGNOSIS AND DSM-IV CRITERIA

The diagnostic criteria for **specific phobias** is as follows:

1. Persistent excessive fear brought on by a specific situation or object
2. Exposure to the situation brings about an immediate anxiety response.
3. Patient recognizes that the fear is excessive.
4. The situation is avoided when possible or tolerated with intense anxiety.
5. If person is under age 18, duration must be at least 6 months.

Agoraphobia:
Agora—open place
Phobia—fear

A 35-year-old female complains of a pounding heart, shortness of breath, and sweating that occur when she takes the train to work. She states that these symptoms also occur when she is in crowded waiting areas. She has decided to avoid the train and get a ride from her friend to work. *Think: Panic disorder with agorophobia.*

Common Specific Phobias
- Fear of animals
- Fear of heights
- Fear of blood or needles
- Fear of illness or injury
- Fear of death
- Fear of flying

Common Social Phobias
- Speaking in public
- Eating in public
- Using public restrooms

A 32-year-old construction worker states that he is terrified of heights. He came in to your office because he recently started a project on the 50th floor and has had trouble doing his job. *Think: Specific phobia.*

Substance-related disorders are found more commonly in phobic patients, especially alcohol-related disorders. Up to one third of phobic patients also have associated major depression.

A 20-year-old college student has always felt "shy" and avoids answering questions in her literature class. Last Monday, she stayed home although she had to give a speech in class, because she did not want to make a "fool out of herself" in front of her classmates. *Think: Social phobia.*

The diagnosis of **social phobia** has the same criteria as above except that the feared situation is related to social settings in which the patient might be embarrassed or humiliated in front of other people.

EPIDEMIOLOGY

Phobias are **the most common mental disorders** in the United States. At least 5 to 10% of the population is afflicted with a phobic disorder, and some studies report as high as 25% of the population. The diagnosis of specific phobia is more common than social phobia. Onset can be as early as 5 years old for phobias such as seeing blood, and as old as 35 for situational fears (such as a fear of heights). The average age of onset for social phobias is mid-teens.

Women are two times as likely to have specific phobia as men; social phobia occurs equally in men and women.

ETIOLOGY

The cause of phobias is most likely multifactorial, with the following components playing important parts:
- *Genetic:* Fear of seeing blood often runs in families and may be associated with an inherited, exaggerated vasovagal response. First-degree relatives of patients with social phobia are three times more likely to develop the disorder.
- *Behavioral:* Phobias may develop through association with traumatic events. For example, people who were in a car accident may develop a specific phobia for driving.
- *Neurochemical:* An overproduction of adrenergic neurotransmitters may contribute to anxiety symptoms. This has led to the successful treatment of some phobias. (Most notably, performance anxiety is often successfully treated with beta blockers).

COURSE AND PROGNOSIS

The course and prognosis are not clearly defined due to their recent recognition.

TREATMENT

Specific Phobia
Pharmacological treatment has not been found effective. **Systemic desensitization** (with or without hypnosis) and supportive psychotherapy are often useful. If necessary, a short course of benzodiazepines or beta blockers may be used during desensitization to help control autonomic symptoms.

Systemic desensitization: Gradually expose patient to feared object or situation while teaching relaxation and breathing techniques.

Social Phobia
Paroxetine (Paxil), an SSRI, is FDA approved for the treatment of social anxiety disorder. Beta blockers are frequently used to control symptoms of performance anxiety. Cognitive and behavioral therapies are useful adjuncts.

Obsessive–Compulsive Disorder (OCD)

Obsession—a recurrent and intrusive thought, feeling, or idea

Compulsion—a conscious repetitive behavior linked to an obsession that, when performed, functions to relieves anxiety caused by the obsession

OCD is an Axis I disorder in which patients have recurrent intrusive thoughts (obsessions) that increase their anxiety level. They usually relieve this anxiety with recurrent standardized behaviors (compulsions). Patients are generally aware of their problems and realize that their thoughts and behaviors are irrational (they have *insight*). The symptoms cause significant distress in their lives, and patients wish they could get rid of them (i.e., their obsessions and compulsions are *ego-dystonic*).

OCD can cause significant impairment of daily functioning, as behaviors are often time consuming and interfere with routines, work, and interpersonal relationships.

DIAGNOSIS AND DSM-IV CRITERIA

1. Either obsessions or compulsions as defined below:
    Obsessions
    - Recurrent and persistent intrusive thoughts or impulses that cause marked anxiety and are not simply excessive worries about real problems
    - Person attempts to suppress the thoughts.
    - Person realizes thoughts are product of his or her own mind.

    Compulsions
    - Repetitive behaviors that the person feels driven to perform in response to an obsession
    - The behaviors are aimed at reducing distress, but there is no realistic link between the behavior and the distress.
2. The person is aware that the obsessions and compulsions are unreasonable and excessive.
3. The obsessions cause marked distress, are time consuming, or significantly interfere with daily functioning.

COMMON PATTERNS OF OBSESSIONS AND COMPULSIONS

1. Obsessions about **contamination** followed by excessive washing or compulsive avoidance of the feared contaminant
2. Obsessions of **doubt** (forgetting to turn off the stove, lock the door, etc.) followed by repeated **checking** to avoid potential danger
3. Obsessions about **symmetry** followed by compulsively slow performance of a task (such as eating, showering, etc.)
4. **Intrusive thoughts** with no compulsion. Thoughts are often sexual or violent.

EPIDEMIOLOGY

- Lifetime population prevalence: 2 to 3%
- Onset is usually in early adulthood, and men are equally likely to be affected as women.
- OCD is associated with major depressive disorder, eating disorders, other anxiety disorders, and obsessive–compulsive personality disorder.
- The rate of OCD is higher in patients with first-degree relatives who have *Tourette's disorder*.

A 28-year-old medical student comes to your office because he is distressed by his repetitive checking of the car door to see if it is locked. He states that after he parks the car and gets to his house, he feels as if the car door is not locked and goes back to check on it. This happens several times and has led to his being late for his clerkships and getting yelled at by his chief. *Think: Obsessive–compulsive disorder.*

Seventy-five percent of OCD patients have **both** obsessions and compulsions.

Obsessive–Compulsive Personality Disorder: Don't get this mixed up with OCD! This is a personality disorder (therefore Axis II) in which the person is excessively preoccupied with details, lists, and organization. He or she is overconscientious and inflexible and perceives no problem (symptoms are *ego-syntonic*, and patients lack insight).

Patients with OCD often initially seek help from nonpsychiatric physicians. For example, they may visit a dermatologist complaining of skin problems on their hands (related to their frequent hand washing).

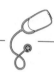

Treatment of OCD often requires *high doses* of SSRIs.

ETIOLOGY

- *Neurochemical:* OCD is associated with abnormal regulation of serotonin.
- *Genetic:* Rates of OCD are higher in first-degree relatives and monozygotic twins than in the general population.
- *Psychosocial:* The onset of OCD is triggered by a stressful life event in approximately 60% of patients.

COURSE AND PROGNOSIS

The course is variable but usually chronic, with only about 30% of patients showing significant improvement with treatment. Forty to 50% of patients have moderate improvement, and 20 to 40% remain significantly impaired or experience worsening of symptoms.

TREATMENT

Pharmacologic
- SSRIs are the first line of treatment, but higher-than-normal doses may be required to be effective.
- Tricyclic antidepressants (TCAs) (clomipramine) are also effective.

Behavioral Treatment
Behavioral therapy is considered as effective as pharmacotherapy in the treatment of OCD; best outcomes are often achieved when both are used simultaneously. The technique, called *exposure and response prevention* (ERP), involves prolonged exposure to the ritual-eliciting stimulus and prevention of the relieving compulsion (e.g., the patient must touch the dirty floor without washing his or her hands). Relaxation techniques are employed to help the patient manage the anxiety that occurs when the compulsion is prevented.

Last Resort
In severe, treatment-resistant cases, electroconvulsive therapy (ECT) or surgery (cingulotomy) may be effective.

Posttraumatic Stress Disorder (PTSD)

PTSD is a response to a catastrophic (life-threatening) life experience in which the patient reexperiences the trauma, avoids reminders of the event, and experiences emotional numbing or hyperarousal.

DIAGNOSIS AND DSM-IV CRITERA

- Having experienced or witnessed a traumatic event (e.g., war, rape, or natural disaster). The event was potentially harmful or fatal, and the initial reaction was intense fear or horror.
- Persistent reexperiencing of the event (e.g., in dreams, flashbacks, or recurrent recollections)
- Avoidance of stimuli associated with the trauma (e.g., avoiding a location that will remind him or her of the event or having difficulty recalling details of the event). *Example:* A woman will not enter parking lots after being raped in one.
- Numbing of responsiveness (limited range of affect, feelings of detachment or estrangement from others, etc.)

- Persistent symptoms of increased arousal (e.g., difficulty sleeping, outbursts of anger, exaggerated startle response, or difficulty concentrating)
- Symptoms must be present for at least 1 month.

COMORBIDITIES

Patients have a high incidence of associated substance abuse and depression.

PROGNOSIS

One half of patients remain symptom free after 3 months of treatment.

TREATMENT

Pharmacological
- TCAs—imipramine and doxepin
- SSRIs, MAOIs
- Anticonvulsants (for flashbacks and nightmares)

Other
- Psychotherapy
- Relaxation training
- Support groups, family therapy

A 23-old-woman who was raped 5 months ago complains of recurrent thoughts of that event every time a coworker touches her. She states this has been happening for the past 2 months often accompanied by nightmares that wake her up at night. She feels extremely anxious when these thoughts "pop in" and lately has had trouble working at her job. *Think: Posttraumatic stress disorder.*

Acute Stress Disorder (ASD)

DIAGNOSIS AND DSM-IV CRITERIA

The diagnosis of acute stress disorder is reserved for patients who experience a major traumatic event but have anxiety symptoms for only a short duration. To qualify for this diagnosis, the symptoms must occur within 1 month of the trauma and last for a maximum of 1 month. Symptoms are similar to those of PTSD.

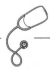

The presence of psychological symptoms after a stressful but *non–life-threatening* event suggests *adjustment disorder* (see below).

PTSD VERSUS ACUTE STRESS DISORDER

PTSD
Event occurred at any time in past
Symptoms last > 1 month

Acute Stress Disorder
Event occurred < 1 month ago
Symptoms last < 1 month

TREATMENT

Same as treatment for PTSD (see above).

Addictive substances (benzodiazepines, etc.) should be avoided (if possible) in the treatment of PTSD because of the high rate of substance abuse in these patients.

Generalized Anxiety Disorder (GAD)

Patients with GAD have persistent, excessive anxiety and hyperarousal for at least 6 months. They worry about general daily events, and their anxiety is difficult to control.

DIAGNOSIS AND DSM-IV CRITERIA

- Excessive anxiety and worry about daily events and activities for at least 6 months

Two weeks after witnessing a car accident in which his friend was killed, a 20-year-old male has stopped going to all his classes and has been extremely anxious. *Think: Acute stress disorder.*

A 36-year-old office clerk states that she constantly wonders if she is capable of doing her job and feels as if she is not good enough. She constantly worries about the mortgage payments, telephone bills, and her children's education. This has been going on over the past few years. *Think: Generalized anxiety disorder.*

"Excessive anxiety" must cause significant distress in the person's life and be present most days of the week for a diagnosis of GAD. The anxiety is *free-floating,* as it does not involve a specific person, event, or activity.

- It is difficult to control the worry.
- Must be associated with at least three of the following:
  - Restlessness
  - Fatigue
  - Difficulty concentrating
  - Irritability
  - Muscle tension
  - Sleep disturbance

EPIDEMIOLOGY

- Lifetime prevalence: 45%
- GAD is very common in the general population.
- Women are two times as likely to have GAD as men.
- Onset is usually before the age of 20; many patients report lifetime of "feeling anxious."

CLINICAL PRESENTATION

Most patients do not initially seek psychiatric help. Most seek out a specialist because of their somatic complaints that accompany this disorder, such as muscle tension or fatigue.

ETIOLOGY

Not completely understood, but biological and psychosocial factors contribute

COMORBIDITIES

Fifty to 90% of patients with GAD have a coexisting mental disorder, especially major depression, social or specific phobia, or panic disorder.

PROGNOSIS

GAD is chronic, with lifelong, fluctuating symptoms in 50% of patients. The other half of patients will fully recover within several years of therapy.

TREATMENT

The most effective treatment approach is a combination of psychotherapy and pharmacotherapy.

Pharmacological
- Buspirone
- Benzodiazepines (usually clonazepam or diazepam)—should be tapered off as soon as possible because of risk of tolerance and dependence
- SSRIs
- Venlafaxine (extended release)

Other
- Behavioral therapy
- Psychotherapy

Adjustment disorders are not considered anxiety disorders. They occur when maladaptive behavioral or emotional symptoms develop after a stressful life event. Symptoms begin within 3 months after the event, end within 6 months, and cause significant impairment in daily functioning or interpersonal relationships.

DIAGNOSIS AND DSM-IV CRITERIA

1. Development of emotional or behavioral symptoms within 3 months after a stressful life event. These symptoms produce either:
   - Severe distress in excess of what would be expected after such an event
   - Significant impairment in daily functioning
2. The symptoms are not those of bereavement.
3. Symptoms resolve within 6 months after stressor has terminated.

Subtypes: Symptoms are coded based on a predominance of either depressed mood, anxiety, disturbance of conduct (such as aggression), or combinations of the above.

EPIDEMIOLOGY

- Adjustment disorders are very common.
- They occur twice as often in females.
- They are most frequently diagnosed in adolescents but may occur at any age.

ETIOLOGY

Triggered by psychosocial factors

PROGNOSIS

May be chronic if the stressor is recurrent; symptoms resolve within 6 months of cessation of stressor (by definition).

TREATMENT

- Supportive psychotherapy (most effective)
- Group therapy
- Pharmacotherapy for associated symptoms (insomnia, anxiety, or depression)

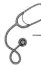

It is important to rule out medical conditions that produce anxiety states such as hyperthyroidism. Ask about caffeine intake.

In adjustment disorder, the stressful event is not life threatening (such as a divorce, death of a loved one, or loss of a job). In PTSD, it is.

HIGH-YIELD FACTS

Anxiety and Adjustment

Personality Disorders

▶ DEFINITION

Personality is one's set of stable, predictable emotional and behavioral traits. Personality *disorders* involve deeply ingrained, inflexible patterns of relating to others that are **maladaptive** and cause significant impairment in social or occupational functioning. Patients with personality disorders lack insight about their problems; their symptoms are **ego-syntonic.** Personality disorders are Axis II diagnoses.

DIAGNOSIS AND DSM-IV CRITERIA

1. Pattern of behavior/inner experience that deviates from the person's culture and is manifested in two or more of the following ways:
   - Cognition
   - Affect
   - Personal relations
   - Impulse control
2. The pattern:
   - Is **pervasive** and **inflexible** in a broad range of situations
   - Is **stable** and has an onset no later than adolescence or early adulthood
   - Leads to significant distress in functioning
   - Is not accounted for by another mental/medical illness or by use of a substance

Each personality disorder is present in 1% of the population. Many patients with personality disorders will meet the criteria for more than one disorder. They should be classified as having all of the disorders for which they qualify.

▶ CLUSTERS

Personality disorders are divided into three clusters:
   Cluster A—schizoid, schizotypal, and paranoid:
   - Patients seem eccentric, peculiar, or withdrawn.
   - Familial association with psychotic disorders

Many people have odd tendencies and quirks; these are not pathological unless they cause significant distress or impairment in daily functioning.

Personality disorder criteria: CAPRI
Cognition
Affect
Personal **R**elations
Impulse control

Personality disorder clusters:
Cluster A: **MAD**
Cluster B: **BAD**
Cluster C: **SAD**

Cluster B—antisocial, borderline, histrionic, and narcissistic:

- Patients seem emotional, dramatic, or inconsistent.
- Familial association with mood disorders

Cluster C—avoidant, dependent, and obsessive–compulsive:

- Patients seem anxious or fearful.
- Familial association with anxiety disorders

Personality disorder not otherwise specified (NOS) includes disorders that do not fit into clusters A, B, or C (including passive–aggressive personality disorder).

ETIOLOGY

Biological, genetic, and psychosocial factors contribute to the development of personality disorders. The prevalence of personality disorders in monozygotic twins is several times higher than in dizygotic twins.

TREATMENT

Personality disorders are generally very difficult to treat, especially since few patients are aware that they need help. The disorders tend to be chronic and lifelong. In general, pharmacologic treatment has limited usefulness (see individual exceptions below) except in treating coexisting symptoms of depression, anxiety, and the like. Psychotherapy and group therapy are usually the most helpful.

> ## ▶ CLUSTER A

Paranoid, **s**chizoid, and **s**chizotypal. These patients are perceived as being eccentric and "weird."

Paranoid Personality Disorder (PPD)

Patients with PPD have a pervasive distrust and suspiciousness of others and often interpret motives as malevolent. They tend to blame their own problems on others and seem angry and hostile.

DIAGNOSIS AND DSM-IV CRITERIA

Diagnosis requires a general distrust of others, beginning by early adulthood and present in a variety of contexts. At least four of the following must also be present:

1. Suspicion (without evidence) that others are exploiting or deceiving him or her
2. Preoccupation with doubts of loyalty or trustworthiness of acquaintances
3. Reluctance to confide in others
4. Interpretation of benign remarks as threatening or demeaning
5. Persistence of grudges
6. Perception of attacks on his or her character that are not apparent to others; quick to counterattack
7. Recurrence of suspicions regarding fidelity of spouse or lover

A 30-year-old male says that his wife has been cheating on him because he does not have a good enough job to provide for her needs. He also claims that on his previous job, his boss laid him off because he did a better job than his boss. *Think: Paranoid personality disorder.*

EPIDEMIOLOGY

- Prevalence: 0.5 to 2.5%
- Men are more likely to have PPD than women.
- Higher incidence in family members of schizophrenics

DIFFERENTIAL DIAGNOSIS

Paranoid schizophrenia: Unlike patients with schizophrenia, patients with paranoid personality disorder *do not have any fixed delusions and are not frankly psychotic*, although they may have transient psychosis under stressful situations.

COURSE AND PROGNOSIS

- Some patients with PPD may eventually be diagnosed with schizophrenia.
- The disorder usually has a chronic course, causing lifelong marital and job-related problems.

TREATMENT

Psychotherapy is the treatment of choice. Patients may also benefit from antianxiety medications or short course of antipsychotics for transient psychosis.

Schizoid Personality Disorder

Patients with schizoid personality disorder have a lifelong pattern of social withdrawal. They are often perceived as eccentric and reclusive. They are quiet and unsociable and have a constricted affect. They have *no desire for close relationships* and prefer to be alone.

DIAGNOSIS AND DSM-IV CRITERIA

A pattern of voluntary social withdrawal and restricted range of emotional expression, beginning by early adulthood and present in a variety of contexts. Four or more of the following must also be present:

1. Neither enjoying nor desiring close relationships (including family)
2. Generally choosing solitary activities
3. Little (if any) interest in sexual activity with another person
4. Taking pleasure in few activities (if any)
5. Few close friends or confidants (if any)
6. Indifference to praise or criticism
7. Emotional coldness, detachment, or flattened affect

EPIDEMIOLOGY

- Prevalence: Approximately 7%
- Men are two times as likely to have schizoid personality disorder as women.
- There is not an increased incidence of schizoid personality disorder in families with history of schizophrenia.

DIFFERENTIAL DIAGNOSIS

- *Paranoid schizophrenia:* Unlike patients with schizophrenia, patients with schizoid personality disorder do not have any fixed delusions, although these may exist transiently in some patients.

Unlike with avoidant personality disorder, patients with schizoid personality disorder *prefer to be alone.*

A 45-year-old scientist works in the lab most of the day and has no friends, according to his coworkers. He expresses no desire to make friends and is content with his single life. He has no evidence of a thought disorder. *Think: Schizoid personality disorder.*

- *Schizoid is an android.*
- *Schizotypical bit the Bible.*

- *Schizotypal personality disorder:* Patients with schizoid personality disorder do not have the same eccentric behavior or magical thinking seen in patients with schizotypal personality disorder.

COURSE

Usually chronic course, but not always lifelong

TREATMENT

Similar to paranoid personality disorder:
- Psychotherapy is the treatment of choice; group therapy is often beneficial.
- Low-dose antipsychotics (short course) if transiently psychotic, or anti-depressants if comorbid major depression is diagnosed

Schizotypal Personality Disorder

Patients with schizotypal personality disorder have a pervasive pattern of eccentric behavior and peculiar thought patterns. They are often perceived as strange and eccentric.

DIAGNOSIS AND DSM-IV CRITERIA

A pattern of social deficits marked by eccentric behavior, cognitive or perceptual distortions, and discomfort with close relationships, beginning by early adulthood and present in a variety of contexts. Five or more of the following must be present:

1. Ideas of reference (excluding delusions of reference)
2. Odd beliefs or magical thinking, inconsistent with cultural norms
3. Unusual perceptual experiences (such as bodily illusions)
4. Suspiciousness
5. Inappropriate or restricted affect
6. Odd or eccentric appearance or behavior
7. Few close friends or confidants
8. Odd thinking or speech (vague, stereotyped, etc.)
9. Excessive social anxiety

A 35-year-old man dresses in a space suit every Tuesday and Thursday. He has computers set up in his basement to "detect the precise time of alien invasion." He has no evidence of auditory or visual hallucinations. *Think: Schizotypal personality disorder.*

Magical thinking may include:
- Belief in clairvoyance or telepathy
- Bizarre fantasies or preoccupations
- Belief in superstitions

Odd behaviors may include involvement in cults or strange religious practices.

EPIDEMIOLOGY

- Prevalence: 3.0%
- More prevalent in monozygotic than dizygotic twins

DIFFERENTIAL DIAGNOSIS

- *Paranoid schizophrenia:* Unlike patients with schizophrenia, patients with schizotypal personality disorder are not frankly psychotic (though they can become transiently so under stress).
- *Schizoid personality disorder:* Patients with schizoid personality disorder do not have the same eccentric behavior seen in patients with schizotypal personality disorder.

COURSE

Course is chronic or patients may eventually develop schizophrenia.

TREATMENT

- Psychotherapy is the treatment of choice.
- Short course of low-dose antipsychotics if necessary (for transient psychosis)

Includes antisocial, borderline, histrionic, and narcissistic personality disorders. These patients are often emotional, impulsive, and dramatic.

Antisocial Personality Disorder

Patients diagnosed with antisocial personality disorder refuse to conform to social norms and lack remorse for their actions. They are impulsive, deceitful, and often violate the law. However, they often appear charming and normal to others who meet them for the first time and do not know their history.

DIAGNOSIS AND DSM-IV CRITERIA

Pattern of disregard for others and violation of the rights of others since age 15. Patients must be **at least 18 years old** for this diagnosis; history of behavior as a child/adolescent must be consistent with **conduct disorder** (see chapter on Psychiatric Disorders in Children). Three or more of the following should be present:

1. Failure to conform to social norms by committing unlawful acts
2. Deceitfulness/repeated lying/manipulating others for personal gain
3. Impulsivity/failure to plan ahead
4. Irritability and aggressiveness/repeated fights or assaults
5. Recklessness and disregard for safety of self or others
6. Irresponsibility/failure to sustain work or honor financial obligations
7. Lack of remorse for actions

EPIDEMIOLOGY

- Prevalence: 3% in men and 1% in women
- Higher incidence in poor urban areas and in prisoners
- Genetic component: Five times increased risk among first-degree relatives

DIFFERENTIAL DIAGNOSIS

Drug abuse: It is necessary to ascertain which came first. Patients who began abusing drugs before their antisocial behavior started may have behavior attributable to the effects of their addiction.

COURSE

Usually has a chronic course, but some improvement of symptoms may occur as the patient ages. Many patients have multiple somatic complaints, and co-existence of substance abuse and/or major depression is common.

Antisocial personality disorder begins in childhood as **conduct disorder.** Patient may have a history of being abused (physically or sexually) as a child or a history of hurting animals or starting fires. It is often associated with violations of the law.

A 30-year-old unemployed male has been accused of killing three senior citizens after robbing them. He is surprisingly charming in the interview. In his adolescence, he was arrested several times for stealing cars and assaulting other kids. *Think: Antisocial personality disorder.*

Borderline personality: IMPULSIVE
Impulsive
Moody
Paranoid under stress
Unstable self image
Labile, intense relationships
Suicidal
Inappropriate anger
Vulnerable to abandonment
Emptiness

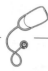

The name *borderline* comes from the patient's being on the borderline of neurosis and psychosis.

A 23-year-old medical student attempted to slit her wrist because things did not work out with a guy she was going out with over the past 3 weeks. She states that guys are jerks and "not worth her time." She often feels that she is "alone in this world." *Think: Borderline personality disorder.*

Patients commonly use defense mechanism of *splitting*—they view others as all good or all bad. (Clinical example: "You are the only doctor who has ever helped me. Every doctor I met before you was horrible.")

TREATMENT

Psychotherapy is the treatment of choice. Pharmacotherapy may be used to treat symptoms of anxiety or depression, but use caution due to high addictive potential of these patients.

Borderline Personality Disorder (BPD)

Patients with BPD have unstable moods, behaviors, and interpersonal relationships. They feel alone in the world and have problems with self-image. They are impulsive and may have a history of repeated suicide attempts/gestures or episodes of self-mutilation.

DIAGNOSIS AND DSM-IV CRITERIA

Pervasive pattern of impulsivity and unstable relationships, affects, self-image, and behaviors, present by early adulthood and in a variety of contexts. At least five of the following must be present:

1. Desperate efforts to avoid real or imagined abandonment
2. Unstable, intense interpersonal relationships
3. Unstable self-image
4. Impulsivity in at least two potentially harmful ways (spending, sexual activity, substance use, etc.)
5. Recurrent suicidal threats or attempts or self-mutilation
6. Unstable mood/affect
7. General feeling of emptiness
8. Difficulty controlling anger
9. Transient, stress-related paranoid ideation or dissociative symptoms

EPIDEMIOLOGY

- Prevalence: 1 to 2%
- Women are two times as likely to have BPD as men.
- 10% suicide rate

DIFFERENTIAL DIAGNOSIS

Schizophrenia: Unlike patients with schizophrenia, patients with borderline personality disorder do not have frank psychosis (may have transient psychosis, however, if decompensate under stress).

COURSE

Usually has a stable, chronic course. High incidence of coexisting major depression and/or substance abuse; increased risk of suicide (often because patients will make suicide gestures and kill themselves by accident).

TREATMENT

- Psychotherapy is the treatment of choice—behavior therapy, cognitive therapy, social skills training, and the like.
- Pharmacotherapy to treat psychotic or depressive symptoms as necessary

Histrionic Personality Disorder (HPD)

Patients with HPD exhibit attention-seeking behavior and excessive emotionality. They are dramatic, flamboyant, and extroverted but are unable to form long-lasting, meaningful relationships. They are often sexually inappropriate and provocative.

DIAGNOSIS AND DSM-IV CRITERIA

Pattern of excessive emotionality and attention seeking, present by early adulthood and in a variety of contexts. At least five of the following must be present:

1. Uncomfortable when not the center of attention
2. Inappropriately seductive or provocative behavior
3. Uses physical appearance to draw attention to self
4. Has speech that is impressionistic and lacking in detail
5. Theatrical and exaggerated expression of emotion
6. Easily influenced by others or situation
7. Perceives relationships as more intimate than they actually are

EPIDEMIOLOGY

- Prevalence: 2 to 3%
- Women are more likely to have HPD than men.

DIFFERENTIAL DIAGNOSIS

Borderline personality disorder: Patients with BPD are more likely to suffer from depression and to attempt suicide. HPD patients are generally more functional.

COURSE

Usually has a chronic course, with some improvement of symptoms with age

TREATMENT

- Psychotherapy is the treatment of choice.
- Pharmacotherapy to treat associated depressive or anxious symptoms as necessary

Narcissistic Personality Disorder (NPD)

Patients with NPD have a sense of superiority, a need for admiration, and a lack of empathy. They consider themselves "special" and will exploit others for their own gain. Despite their grandiosity, however, these patients often have fragile self-esteems.

DIAGNOSIS AND DSM-IV CRITERIA

Pattern of grandiosity, need for admiration, and lack of empathy beginning by early adulthood and present in a variety of contexts. Five or more of the following must be present:

1. Exaggerated sense of self-importance
2. Preoccupied with fantasies of unlimited money, success, brilliance, etc.
3. Believes that he or she is "special" or unique and can associate only with other high-status individuals
4. Needs excessive admiration
5. Has sense of entitlement
6. Takes advantage of others for self-gain

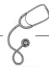

Pharmacotherapy has been shown to be more useful in borderline personality disorder than in any other personality disorder.

Histrionic patients often use defense mechanism of *regression*—they revert to childlike behaviors.

A 33-year-old scantily clad woman comes to your office complaining that her fever feels like "she is burning in hell." She vividly describes how the fever has affected her work as a teacher. *Think: Histrionic personality disorder.*

A 48-year-old company CEO is rushed to the ED after an automobile accident. He does not let the residents operate on him and requests the Chief of Trauma Surgery because he is "vital to the company." He makes several business phone calls in the ED to stay on "top of his game." *Think: Narcissistic personality disorder.*

7. Lacks empathy
8. Envious of others or believes others are envious of him or her
9. Arrogant or haughty

EPIDEMIOLOGY

Prevalence: < 1%

DIFFERENTIAL DIAGNOSIS

Antisocial personality disorder: Both types of patients exploit others, but NPD patients want status and recognition, while antisocial patients want material gain or simply the subjugation of others. Narcissistic patients become depressed when they don't get the recognition they think they deserve.

COURSE

Usually has a chronic course; higher incidence of depression and midlife crises since these patients put such a high value on youth and power.

TREATMENT

- Psychotherapy is the treatment of choice.
- Antidepressants or lithium may be used as needed (for mood swings if a comorbid mood disorder is diagnosed).

▶ CLUSTER C

Includes avoidant, dependent, and obsessive–compulsive personality disorders. These patients appear anxious and fearful.

Avoidant Personality Disorder

Patients with avoidant personality disorder have a pervasive pattern of social inhibition and an intense fear of rejection. They will avoid situations in which they may be rejected. Their fear of rejection is so overwhelming that it affects all aspects of their lives. They avoid social interactions and seek jobs in which there is little interpersonal contact. These patients *desire* companionship but are extremely shy and easily injured.

DIAGNOSIS AND DSM-IV CRITERIA

A pattern of social inhibition, hypersensitivity, and feelings of inadequacy since early adulthood, with at least four of the following:

1. Avoids occupation that involves interpersonal contact due to a fear of criticism and rejection
2. Unwilling to interact unless certain of being liked
3. Cautious of intrapersonal relationships
4. Preoccupied with being criticized or rejected in social situations
5. Inhibited in new social situations because he or she feels inadequate
6. Believes he or she is socially inept and inferior
7. Reluctant to engage in new activities for fear of embarrassment

A 30-year-old postal worker rarely goes out with her coworkers and often makes excuses when they ask her to join them because she is afraid they will not like her. She wishes to go out and meet new people but according to her, she is too "shy." *Think: Avoidant personality disorder.*

EPIDEMIOLOGY

- Prevalence: 1 to 10%
- Sex ratio not known

DIFFERENTIAL DIAGNOSIS

Schizoid personality disorder: Patients with avoidant personality disorder desire companionship but are extremely shy, whereas patients with schizoid personality disorder have no desire for companionship.

Social phobia (social anxiety disorder): See chapter on Anxiety and Adjustment Disorders. Both disorders involve fear and avoidance of social situations. If the symptoms are an integral part of the patient's personality and have been evident since before adulthood, personality disorder is the more likely diagnosis. Social phobia involves a fear of *embarrassment* in a particular setting (speaking in public, urinating in public, etc.), whereas avoidant personality disorder is an overall fear of *rejection* and a sense of inadequacy. However, a patient can have both disorders concurrently and should carry both diagnoses if criteria for each are met.

Dependent personality disorder: Avoidant personality disorder patients cling to relationships, similar to dependent personality disorder patients; however, avoidant patients are slow to get involved, whereas dependents actively and aggressively seek relationships.

Schizoid patients *prefer* to be alone. Avoidant patients want to be with others but are too scared of rejection.

COURSE

- Course is usually chronic.
- Particularly difficult during adolescence, when attractiveness and socialization are important
- Increased incidence of associated anxiety and depressive disorders

TREATMENT

- Psychotherapy, including assertiveness training, is most effective.
- Beta blockers may be used to control autonomic symptoms of anxiety, and selective serotonin reuptake inhibitors (SSRIs) may be prescribed for major depression.

Dependent Personality Disorder (DPD)

Patients with DPD have poor self-confidence and fear separation. They have an excessive need to be taken care of and allow others to make decisions for them. They feel helpless when left alone.

DIAGNOSIS AND DSM-IV CRITERIA

A pattern of submissive and clinging behavior due to excessive need to be taken care of. At least five of the following must be present:

1. Difficulty making everyday decisions without reassurance from others
2. Needs others to assume responsibilities for most areas of his or her life
3. Cannot express disagreement because of fear of loss of approval
4. Difficulty initiating projects because of lack of self-confidence
5. Goes to excessive lengths to obtain support from others
6. Feels helpless when alone
7. Urgently seeks another relationship when one ends
8. Preoccupied with fears of being left to take care of self

A 40-year-old man who lives with his parents has trouble deciding on how to go about having his car fixed. He calls his father at work several times to ask very trivial things. He has been unemployed over the past 3 years. *Think: Dependent personality disorder.*

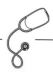

Many people with debilitating illnesses can develop dependent traits. However, to be diagnosed with DPD, the features must manifest before early adulthood.

EPIDEMIOLOGY

- Prevalence: Approximately 1%
- Women are more likely to have DPD than men.

DIFFERENTIAL DIAGNOSIS

- *Avoidant personality disorder:* See discussion above.
- *Borderline and histrionic personality disorder:* Patients with DPD usually have a long-lasting relationship with one person on whom they are dependent. Patients with borderline and histrionic personality disorders are often dependent on other people, but they are unable to maintain a long-lasting relationship.

COURSE

- Usually has a chronic course
- Often, symptoms decrease with age and/or with therapy.
- Patients are prone to depression, particularly after loss of person on whom they are dependent.

TREATMENT

- Psychotherapy is the treatment of choice.
- Pharmacotherapy may be used to treat associated symptoms of anxiety or depression.

Obsessive–Compulsive Personality Disorder (OCPD)

Patients with OCPD have a pervasive pattern of perfectionism, inflexibility, and orderliness. They get so preoccupied with unimportant details that they are often unable to complete simple tasks in a timely fashion. They appear stiff, serious, and formal with constricted affect. They are often successful professionally but have poor interpersonal skills.

A 40-year-old secretary has been recently fired because of her inability to prepare some work projects in time. According to her, they were not in the right format and she had to revise them six times, which led to the delay. This has happened before but she feels that she is not given enough time. *Think: Obsessive–compulsive personality disorder.*

DIAGNOSIS AND DSM-IV CRITERIA

Pattern of preoccupation with orderliness, control, and perfectionism at the expense of efficiency, present by early adulthood and in a variety of contexts. At least four of the following must be present:

1. Preoccupation with details, rules, lists, and organization such that the major point of the activity is lost
2. Perfectionism that is detrimental to completion of task
3. Excessive devotion to work
4. Excessive conscientiousness and scrupulousness about morals and ethics
5. Will not delegate tasks
6. Unable to discard worthless objects
7. Miserly
8. Rigid and stubborn

EPIDEMIOLOGY

- Prevalence unknown
- Men are more likely to have OCPD than women.
- Occurs most often in the oldest child
- Increased incidence in first-degree relatives

- *Obsessive–compulsive disorder (OCD)*: Patients with OCPD do not have the recurrent obsessions or compulsions that are present in obsessive–compulsive disorder. In addition, the symptoms of OCPD are **ego-syntonic** rather than ego-dystonic (as in OCD). That is, OCD patients are aware that they have a problem and wish that their thoughts and behaviors would go away.
- *Narcissistic personality disorder*: Both personalities involve assertiveness and achievement, but NPD patients are motivated by status, whereas OCD patients are motivated by the work itself.

COURSE

- Unpredictable course
- Some patients later develop obsessions or compulsions (OCD), some develop schizophrenia or major depressive disorder, and others may improve or remain stable.

TREATMENT

- Psychotherapy is the treatment of choice. Group therapy and behavior therapy may be useful.
- Pharmacotherapy may be used to treat associated symptoms as necessary.

▶ **PERSONALITY DISORDER NOT OTHERWISE SPECIFIED (NOS)**

This diagnosis is reserved for personality disorders that do not fit into categories A, B, or C. It includes passive–aggressive personality disorder, depressive personality disorder, sadomasochistic personality disorder, and sadistic personality disorder. Only passive–aggressive personality disorder will be discussed briefly here.

Passive–Aggressive Personality Disorder

Passive–aggressive personality disorder was once a separate personality disorder like those listed above but was relegated to the NOS category when DSM-IV was published. Patients with this disorder are stubborn, inefficient procrastinators. They alternate between compliance and defiance and passively resist fulfillment of tasks. They frequently make excuses for themselves and lack assertiveness. They attempt to manipulate others to do their chores, errands, and the like, and frequently complain about their own misfortunes. Psychotherapy is the treatment of choice.

An overweight woman starts a diet, loses 5 pounds, and then says she's taking a "break" from the diet because she "hasn't been feeling well." *Think: passive–aggressive personality disorder.*

HIGH-YIELD FACTS

Personality Disorders

Substance-Related Disorders

► **SUBSTANCE ABUSE**

DIAGNOSIS AND DSM-IV CRITERIA

Abuse is a pattern of substance use leading to impairment or distress for at least 1 year with one or more of the following manifestations:

1. Failure to fulfill obligations at work, school, or home
2. Use in dangerous situations (i.e., driving a car)
3. Recurrent substance-related legal problems
4. Continued use despite social or interpersonal problems due to the substance use

> Know how to distinguish substance abuse from dependence.

► **SUBSTANCE DEPENDENCE**

DIAGNOSIS AND DSM-IV CRITERIA

Dependence is substance use leading to impairment or distress manifested by at least three of the following within a 12-month period:

1. Tolerance (see definition below)
2. Withdrawal (see definition below)
3. Using substance more than originally intended
4. Persistent desire or unsuccessful efforts to cut down on use
5. Significant time spent in getting, using, or recovering from substance
6. Decreased social, occupational, or recreational activities because of substance use
7. Continued use despite subsequent physical or psychological problem (e.g., drinking despite worsening liver problems)

A diagnosis of substance dependence supercedes a diagnosis of substance abuse.

> *Addiction* is not considered a scientific term. Instead, use the word *dependence* when appropriate.

EPIDEMIOLOGY

- Lifetime prevalence of substance abuse or dependence in the United States: Approximately 17%
- More common in men than women

- Caffeine, alcohol, and nicotine are the most commonly used substances.
- Depressive symptoms are common among persons with substance abuse or dependence.

WITHDRAWAL AND TOLERANCE

Withdrawal

The development of a substance-specific syndrome due to the cessation of substance use that has been heavy and prolonged

Tolerance

The need for increased amounts of the substance to achieve the desired effect *or* diminished effect if using the same amount of the substance

▶ ACUTE INTOXICATION AND WITHDRAWAL

The intoxicated patient, or one experiencing withdrawal, can present several problems in both diagnosis and treatment. Since it is common for addicts to abuse several drugs at once, the clinical presentation is often confusing, and signs/symptoms may be atypical; always be on the lookout for polysubstance abuse.

▶ ALCOHOL (EtOH)

Alcohol activates gamma-aminobutyric acid (GABA) and serotonin receptors in the central nervous system (CNS) and inhibits glutamate receptors. GABA receptors are inhibitory, and thus alcohol has a sedating effect.

Alcohol is the most commonly abused substance in the United States. Seven to 10% of Americans are alcoholics.

METABOLISM

Alcohol is metabolized in the following manner:

1. Alcohol → acetaldehyde (enzyme: *alcohol dehydrogenase*)
2. Acetaldehyde → acetic acid (enzyme: *aldehyde dehydrogenase*)

There is upregulation of these enzymes in heavy drinkers. Asian people often have less aldehyde dehydrogenase; the resultant buildup of acetaldehyde causes flushing and nausea.

SCREENING FOR ABUSE

The **CAGE questionnaire** is used to screen for alcohol abuse. Two or more "yes" answers are considered a positive screen; one "yes" answer should arouse suspicion of abuse:

1. Have you ever wanted to **c**ut down on your drinking?
2. Have you ever felt **a**nnoyed by criticism of your drinking?
3. Have you ever felt **g**uilty about drinking?
4. Have you ever taken a drink as an "**e**ye opener" (to prevent the shakes)?

Alcohol is the most common co-ingestant in drug overdoses.

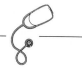

Use the CAGE questionnaire to screen for EtOH abuse.

Alcohol Intoxication

The absorption and elimination rates of alcohol are variable and depend on many factors, including age, sex, body weight, speed of consumption, the presence of food in the stomach, chronic alcoholism, the presence of advanced cirrhosis, and the state of nutrition.

In addition to the above factors, the effects of EtOH also depend on the blood alcohol level (BAL). The values in the following table refer to the BALs of the novice drinker rather than the chronic alcoholic. This is because the latter generate a tolerance to the effects of EtOH and, therefore, may not experience a given effect until the BAL is significantly higher. In most states, the legal limit for intoxication is 80 to 100 mg/dL.

More than 50% of adults with BAL > 150 mg/dL (0.15 mg%) show obvious signs of intoxication.

CLINICAL PRESENTATION

Effects	BAL
Decreased fine motor control	20–50 mg/dL
Impaired judgment and coordination	50–100 mg/dL
Ataxic gait and poor balance	100–150 mg/dL
Lethargy; difficulty sitting upright	150–250 mg/dL
Coma in the novice drinker	300 mg/dL
Respiratory depression	400 mg/dL

DIFFERENTIAL DIAGNOSIS

Hypoglycemia, hypoxia, mixed EtOH–drug overdose, ethylene glycol or methanol poisoning, hepatic encephalopathy, psychosis, and psychomotor seizures

DIAGNOSTIC EVALUATION

Serum EtOH level or an expired air breathalyzer can determine the extent of intoxication. A computed tomographic (CT) scan of the head may be necessary to rule out subdural hematoma or other brain injury.

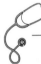

Recall that methanol, ethanol, and ethylene glycol can each cause metabolic acidosis with increased anion gap.

TREATMENT

Intoxication (Acute)

- Ensure adequate airway, breathing, and circulation. Monitor electrolytes and acid–base status.
- Obtain finger-stick glucose level to exclude hypoglycemia.
- **Thiamine** (to prevent or treat Wernicke's encephalopathy), **naloxone** (to reverse the effects of any opioids that may have been ingested), and folate are also administered.

The liver will eventually metabolize alcohol without any other interventions provided that a reliable airway is maintained; a severely intoxicated patient may require intubation while he or she is recovering.

Gastrointestinal evacuation (e.g., gastric lavage and charcoal) has no role in the treatment of EtOH overdose but may be used in mixed EtOH–drug overdose.

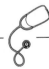

Thiamine, glucose, and naloxone should be given to patients who present with altered mental status.

Dependence (Long Term)

1. Alcoholics Anonymous—self-help group
2. Disulfiram (Antabuse)—aversive therapy; inhibits aldehyde dehydrogenase, causing violent retching when the person drinks
3. Psychotherapy and selective serotonin reuptake inhibitors (SSRIs)
4. Naltrexone—though an opioid antagonist, helps reduce cravings for EtOH

Alcohol Withdrawal

The pathophysiology of the alcohol withdrawal syndrome is poorly understood but is related to the chronic depressant effect of EtOH on the central nervous system. When long-term EtOH consumption ceases, the depressant effect is terminated, and CNS excitation occurs.

CLINICAL PRESENTATION

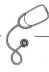

EtOH withdrawal symptoms usually begin in 6 to 24 hours and last 2 to 7 days.
Mild: Irritability, tremor, insomnia
Moderate: Diaphoresis, fever, disorientation
Severe: Grand mal seizures, DTs

The earliest symptoms of EtOH withdrawal begin between 6 and 24 hours after the patient's last drink and depend on the duration and quantity of EtOH consumption. Patients experiencing mild withdrawal may be irritable and complain of insomnia. Those in more severe withdrawal may experience fever, disorientation, seizures, or hallucinations.

The signs and symptoms of the **alcohol withdrawal syndrome** include insomnia, anxiety, tremor, irritability, anorexia, tachycardia, hyperreflexia, hypertension, fever, seizures, hallucinations, and delirium.

Delirium tremens (DTs) is the most serious form of EtOH withdrawal and often begins within 72 hours of cessation of drinking. While only 5% of patients hospitalized for EtOH withdrawal develop DTs, there is a roughly 15 to 20% mortality rate if left untreated. In addition to delirium, symptoms of DTs may include visual or tactile hallucinations, gross tremor, autonomic instability, and fluctuating levels of psychomotor activity.

DIAGNOSTIC EVALUATION

Delirium tremens carries a 15 to 20% mortality rate but occurs in only 5% of patients that are hospitalized for EtOH withdrawal. It is a medical emergency and should be treated with adequate doses of benzodiazepines.

Accurate and frequent assessment of vital signs is essential, as autonomic instability may occur in cases of severe withdrawal and DTs. Careful attention must be given to the level of consciousness, and the possibility of trauma should be investigated. Signs of hepatic failure (e.g., ascites, jaundice, caput medusae, coagulopathy) may be present.

DIFFERENTIAL DIAGNOSIS

Alcohol-induced hypoglycemia, acute schizophrenia, drug-induced psychosis, encephalitis, thyrotoxicosis, anticholinergic poisoning, and withdrawal from other sedative–hypnotic type drugs

TREATMENT

- Tapering doses of benzodiazepines (chlordiazepoxide, lorazepam)
- Thiamine, folic acid, and a multivitamin to treat nutritional deficiencies
- Magnesium sulfate for postwithdrawal seizures

Long-Term Complications of Alcohol Intake

Wernicke–Korsakoff syndrome is caused by thiamine (vitamin B_1) deficiency resulting from the poor diet of alcoholics. **Wernicke's encephalopathy** is acute and can be reversed with thiamine therapy:

1. Ataxia
2. Confusion
3. Ocular abnormalities (nystagmus, gaze palsies)

If left untreated, Wernicke's encephalopathy may progress into **Korsakoff's syndrome,** which is chronic and often irreversible.

1. Impaired recent memory
2. Anterograde amnesia
3. +/– Confabulation

Confabulation: Making up answers when memory has failed

All patients with altered mental status should be given thiamine *before* glucose or Wernicke–Korsakoff syndrome may be precipitated. Thiamine is a coenzyme used in carbohydrate metabolism.

▶ COCAINE

Cocaine blocks dopamine reuptake from the synaptic cleft, causing a stimulant effect. Dopamine plays a role in behavioral reinforcement ("reward" system of the brain).

Cocaine Intoxication

CLINICAL PRESENTATION

Cocaine intoxication often produces euphoria, increased or decreased blood pressure, tachycardia or bradycardia, nausea, dilated pupils, weight loss, psychomotor agitation or depression, chills, and sweating. It may also cause respiratory depression, seizures, arrhythmias, and hallucinations (especially tactile). Since cocaine is an indirect sympathomimetic, intoxication mimics the fight-or-flight response.

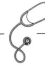

Cocaine overdose can cause death secondary to cardiac arrhythmia, seizure, or respiratory depression.

Cocaine's vasoconstrictive effect may result in myocardial infarction (MI) or cerebrovascular accident (CVA).

DIFFERENTIAL DIAGNOSIS

Amphetamine or phencyclidine (PCP) intoxication, sedative withdrawal

DIAGNOSTIC EVALUATION

Urine drug screen (positive for 3 days, longer in heavy users)

TREATMENT

Intoxication

1. For mild-to-moderate agitation: Benzodiazepines
2. For severe agitation or psychosis: Haloperidol
3. Symptomatic support (i.e., control hypertension, arrhythmias)

Dependence

1. Psychotherapy, group therapy
2. Tricyclic antidepressants (TCAs)
3. Dopamine agonists (amantadine, bromocriptine)

Cocaine Withdrawal

Abrupt abstinence is not life threatening but produces a dysphoric "crash": malaise, fatigue, depression, hunger, constricted pupils, vivid dreams, psychomotor agitation or retardation

TREATMENT

Usually supportive—let patient sleep off crash.

▶ AMPHETAMINES

> *Classic amphetamines:* Dextroamphetamine (Dexedrine), methylphenidate (Ritalin), methamphetamine (Desoxyn, ice, speed, "crystal meth," "crack")
>
> *Substituted ("designer") amphetamines:* MDMA (ecstasy), MDEA (eve)

Classic amphetamines release dopamine from nerve endings, causing a stimulant effect. They are used medically in the treatment of narcolepsy, attention deficit hyperactivity disorder (ADHD), and depressive disorders. *Designer* amphetamines release dopamine and serotonin from nerve endings and have both stimulant and hallucinogenic properties.

Amphetamine Intoxication

CLINICAL PRESENTATION

Amphetamine intoxication causes symptoms similar to those of cocaine (see above).

DIFFERENTIAL DIAGNOSIS

Cocaine or PCP intoxication. Chronic use in high doses may cause a psychotic state that is similar to schizophrenia.

DIAGNOSTIC EVALUATION

Urine drug screen (positive for 1 to 2 days). A negative routine drug screen does not rule out amphetamine use, since most assays are not of adequate sensitivity. A negative drug screen can never completely rule out substance abuse or dependence.

TREATMENT

Similar to cocaine (see above)

Amphetamine Withdrawal

Similar to cocaine withdrawal (see above)

PCP, or "angel dust," is a hallucinogen that antagonizes N-methyl-D-aspartate (NMDA) glutamate receptors and activates dopaminergic neurons. Ketamine is similar to PCP. Both were developed as anesthetic agents.

PCP Intoxication

Intoxication with PCP causes recklessness, impulsiveness, impaired judgment, assaultiveness, rotatory **nystagmus,** ataxia, hypertension, tachycardia, muscle rigidity, and high tolerance to pain. Overdose can cause seizures or coma.

Rotatory nystagmus is pathognomonic for PCP intoxicaton.

TREATMENT

- Monitor blood pressure, temperature, and electrolytes.
- Acidify urine with ammonium chloride and ascorbic acid.
- Benzodiazepines or dopamine antagonists to control agitation and anxiety
- Diazepam for muscle spasms and seizures
- Haloperidol to control severe agitation or psychotic symptoms

More than with other drugs, intoxication with PCP results in violence.

DIFFERENTIAL DIAGNOSIS

Acute psychotic states, schizophrenia

DIAGNOSTIC EVALUATION

Urine drug screen (positive for > 1 week). Creatine phosphokinase (CPK) and aspartate aminotransferase (AST) are often elevated.

PCP Withdrawal

No withdrawal syndrome, but "flashbacks" may occur

These drugs are highly abused in the United States since they are more readily available than other drugs such as cocaine or opioids. *Benzodiazepines* (BDZs) are commonly used in the treatment of anxiety disorders and are therefore obtained easily via prescription. They potentiate the effects of GABA by increasing the frequency of chloride channel opening. *Barbiturates* are used in the treatment of epilepsy and as anesthetics, and they potentiate the effects of GABA by increasing the duration of chloride channel opening. At high doses they act as direct GABA agonists and have a lower margin of safety relative to BDZs. In combination BDZs and barbiturates are synergistic due to their complementary effect on GABA channel opening. Respiratory depression can occur as a complication.

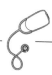

Gamma-hydroxybutyrate (GHB, "Grievous Bodily Harm") is a dose-specific CNS depressant that produces memory loss, respiratory distress, and coma. It is commonly used as a date-rape drug.

Flumazenil is a very short-acting BDZ antagonist. Use with caution when treating overdose, as it may precipitate seizures.

In general, withdrawal from drugs that are sedating is life threatening, while withdrawal from stimulants and hallucinogens is not.

Sedative-Hypnotic Intoxication

Intoxication with sedatives produces drowsiness, slurred speech, incoordination, ataxia, mood lability, impaired judgment, nystagmus, respiratory depression, and coma or death in overdose (especially barbiturates). Symptoms are augmented when combined with EtOH. Long-term sedative use causes dependence.

DIFFERENTIAL DIAGNOSIS

Alcohol intoxication, generalized cerebral dysfunction (i.e., delirium)

DIAGNOSTIC EVALUATION

Urine or serum drug screen (positive for 1 week), electrolytes, electrocardiogram

TREATMENT

- Maintain airway, breathing, and circulation.
- Activated charcoal to prevent further gastrointestinal absorption
- For *barbiturates only:* Alkalinize urine with sodium bicarbonate to promote renal excretion.
- For *benzodiazepines only:* Flumazenil in overdose
- Supportive care—improve respiratory status, control hypotension

Sedative-Hypnotic Withdrawal

Abrupt abstinence after chronic use can be life threatening. While physiological dependence is more likely with short-acting agents, longer-acting agents can also cause withdrawal symptoms.

CLINICAL PRESENTATION

Symptoms of autonomic hyperactivity (tachycardia, sweating, etc.), insomnia, anxiety, tremor, nausea/vomiting, delirium, and hallucinations. Seizures may occur and can be life threatening.

TREATMENT

- Administration of a long-acting benzodiazepine such as chlordiazepoxide or diazepam, with tapering of the dose
- Tegretol or valproic acid may be used for seizure control.

▶ OPIATES

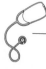

Dextromethorphan is a common ingredient in cough syrup.

Examples: Heroin, codeine, dextromethorphan, morphine, methadone, meperidine (Demerol). These compounds stimulate opiate receptors (mu, kappa, and delta), which are normally stimulated by endogenous opiates and are involved in analgesia, sedation, and dependence. Opiates also have effects on the dopaminergic system, which mediates their addictive and rewarding properties. Endorphins and enkephalins are endogenous opiates.

Opiate Intoxication

Opiate intoxication causes drowsiness, nausea/vomiting, constipation, slurred speech, **constricted pupils,** seizures, and respiratory depression, which may progress to coma or death in overdose.

Meperidine and monoamine oxidase inhibitors taken in combination may cause the **serotonin syndrome:** Hyperthermia, confusion, hyper- or hypotension, and muscular rigidity.

DIFFERENTIAL DIAGNOSIS

Sedative-hypnotic intoxication, severe EtOH intoxication

DIAGNOSTIC EVALUATION

Rapid recovery of consciousness following the administration of intravenous (IV) naloxone (opiate antagonist) is consistent with opiate overdose. Urine and blood tests remain positive for 12 to 36 hours.

TREATMENT

Intoxication
Ensure adequate airway, breathing, and circulation.

Overdose
Administration of naloxone or naltrexone (opiate antagonists) will improve respiratory depression but may cause severe withdrawal in an opiate-dependent patient. Ventilatory support may be required.

Dependence
- Oral methadone once daily, tapered over months to years
- Psychotherapy, support groups (Narcotics Anonymous, etc.)

Opiate Withdrawal

CLINICAL PRESENTATION

While not life threatening, abstinence in the opiate-dependent individual leads to an unpleasant withdrawal syndrome characterized by dysphoria, insomnia, lacrimation, **rhinorrhea,** yawning, weakness, sweating, **piloerection,** nausea/vomiting, fever, dilated pupils, and muscle ache.

TREATMENT

Moderate symptoms: Clonidine and/or buprenorphine
Severe symptoms: Detox with methadone tapered over 7 days.

▶ HALLUCINOGENS

Examples: Psilocybin (mushrooms), mescaline, lysergic acid diethylamide (LSD). Pharmacological effects vary, but LSD is known to act on the serotonergic system. Tolerance to hallucinogens develops quickly but reverses rapidly after cessation. Hallucinogens do not cause physical dependence or withdrawal.

Opiates are naturally occurring chemicals that bind at the opiate receptors. Opioids are synthetic chemicals that bind to these same opiate receptors (e.g., fentanyl)

Classic triad of opioid overdose:
- Respiratory depression
- Altered mental status
- Miosis
"**Rebels Admire Morphine**"

Meperidine is the exception to opioids producing miosis. "Demerol dilates pupils."

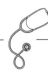

Eating poppy seed bagels or muffins can result in a urine drug screen that is positive for opioids.

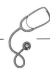

Withdrawal from opiates is *not* life threatening.

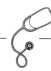

Methyl pemolines ("92C-B," "U4EUH," "Nexus") produce classic psychedelic distortion of senses, including feeling of harmony, anxiety, paranoia, and panic.

Ketamine ("special K") can produce tachycardia and tachypnea with hallucinations at higher doses; also amnesia and numbed confusion.

Hallucinogen Intoxication

Hallucinogens cause perceptual changes, papillary dilation, tachycardia, tremors, incoordination, sweating, and palpitations.

TREATMENT

Guidance and reassurance ("talking down" the patient) are usually enough. In severe cases, antipsychotics or benzodiazepines may be used.

Hallucinogen Withdrawal

No withdrawal syndrome is produced, but patients may experience "flashbacks" later in life (recurrence of symptoms due to reabsorption from lipid stores).

▶ MARIJUANA

The main active component in marijuana, or cannabis, is THC (tetrahydrocannabinol). Cannabinoid receptors in the brain inhibit adenylate cyclase. Effects are increased when used with EtOH.

Marijuana has been shown to successfully treat nausea in cancer patients and to increase appetite in AIDS patients. No dependence or withdrawal syndrome has been shown.

Marijuana Intoxication

Marijuana causes euphoria, impaired coordination, mild tachycardia, **conjunctival injection,** dry mouth, and increased appetite.

Marijuana can be smoked or eaten. Marijuana cigarettes are sometimes dipped in embalming fluid, which causes cognitive dulling as a desired effect.

TREATMENT

Supportive and symptomatic

DIAGNOSTIC EVALUATION

Urine drug screen is positive for up to 4 weeks in heavy users (released from adipose stores).

Marijuana Withdrawal

CLINICAL PRESENTATION

No withdrawal syndrome, but mild irritability, insomnia, nausea, and decreased appetite may occur in heavy users.

TREATMENT

Supportive and symptomatic

Examples: Solvents, glue, paint thinners, fuels, isobutyl nitrates ("rush," "locker room," "bolt"). Inhalants generally act as CNS depressants. User is typically an adolescent male.

Inhalant Intoxication

Inhalants may cause impaired judgment, belligerence, impulsivity, perceptual disturbances, lethargy, dizziness, nystagmus, tremor, muscle weakness, hyporeflexia, ataxia, slurred speech, euphoria, stupor, or coma. Overdose may be fatal secondary to respiratory depression or arrhythmias. Long-term use may cause permanent damage to CNS, peripheral nervous system (PNS), liver, kidney, and muscle.

TREATMENT

- Monitor airway, breathing, and circulation.
- Symptomatic treatment as needed
- Psychotherapy and counseling for dependent patients

DIAGNOSTIC EVALUATION

Serum drug screen (positive for 4 to 10 hours)

Inhalant Withdrawal

A withdrawal syndrome does not usually occur, but symptoms may include irritability, nausea, vomiting, tachycardia, and occasionally hallucinations.

Caffeine is the most commonly used psychoactive substance in the United States, usually in the form of coffee or tea. Caffeine acts as an adenosine antagonist, causing increased cyclic adenosine monophosphate (cAMP) and a stimulant effect via the dopaminergic system.

Caffeine Intoxication

CLINICAL PRESENTATION

Intoxication may occur with consumption of over 250 mg of caffeine. Signs and symptoms include anxiety, insomnia, twitching, rambling speech, flushed face, diuresis, gastrointestinal disturbance, and restlessness. Consumption of more than 1 gram of caffeine may cause tinnitus, severe agitation, and cardiac arrhythmias. In excess of 10 g, death may occur secondary to seizures and respiratory failure.

One cup of coffee: 100 to 150 mg caffeine
One cup of tea: 40 to 60 mg caffeine

TREATMENT

Supportive and symptomatic

Caffeine Withdrawal

Withdrawal symptoms resolve within 1 week and include headache, nausea/vomiting, drowsiness, anxiety, or depression.

TREATMENT

Taper consumption of caffeine-containing products. Use analgesics to treat headaches. Rarely, a short course of benzodiazepines may be indicated to control anxiety.

▶ **NICOTINE**

Nicotine is derived from the tobacco plant and stimulates nicotinic receptors in autonomic ganglia of the sympathetic and parasympathetic nervous systems. Cigarette smoking poses many health risks, and nicotine is rapidly addictive through its effects on the dopaminergic system.

Nicotine Intoxication

Nicotine acts as a CNS stimulant and may cause restlessness, insomnia, anxiety, and increased gastrointestinal motility. Tobacco users report improved attention, improved mood, and decreased tension.

TREATMENT

Cessation

Nicotine Withdrawal

Withdrawal causes intense craving, dysphoria, anxiety, increased appetite, irritability, and insomnia.

TREATMENT

Smoking cessation with the aid of:

1. Behavioral counseling
2. Nicotine replacement therapy (gum, transdermal patch)
3. Zyban—antidepressant that helps reduce cravings
4. Clonidine

Relapse after abstinence is common.

Cigarette smoking during pregnancy is associated with low birth weight and persistent pulmonary hypertension of the newborn.

Cognitive Disorders

▶ DEFINITION

Cognitive disorders affect memory, orientation, attention, and judgment. They result from primary or secondary abnormalities of the central nervous system. The main categories of cognitive disorders are:

- Dementia
- Delirium
- Amnestic disorders

▶ MINI MENTAL STATE EXAM (MMSE)

The MMSE is used to assess a patient's current state of cognitive functioning. It can be used as a daily barometer to evaluate interval changes but should not be used to make a formal diagnosis. It tests orientation, registration, attention and calculation, recall, and language (Table 8-1).

MMSE scoring:
- Perfect score: 30
- Dysfunction: < 25

▶ DEMENTIA

Dementia is an impairment of memory and other cognitive functions without alteration in the level of consciousness. Most forms of dementia are progressive and irreversible. Dementia is a major cause of disability in the elderly. It affects memory, cognition, language skills, behavior, and personality.

EPIDEMIOLOGY

- Incidence increases with age.
- Twenty percent of people > age 80 have a severe form of dementia.
- *Associations:* Delusions and hallucinations occur in approximately 30% of demented patients. Affective symptoms, including depression and anxiety, are seen in 40 to 50% of patients. Personality changes are also common.

The ability to distinguish between **dementia** (= **mem**ory impairment) and **delirium** (= sen**sorium** impairment) is essential for both exam questions and clinical practice (see Table 8-2).

TABLE 8-1. Performing the Mini Mental State Exam	
1. Orientation	
What is the date, month, year?	5 points
Where are we (state, city, hospital)?	5 points
2. Registration	
Name three objects and repeat them.	3 points
3. Attention and calculation	
Serial 7s (subtract 7 from 100 and continue subtracting 7 from each answer) or spell "world" backward.	5 points
4. Recall	
Name the three objects above 5 minutes later.	3 points
5. Language	
Name a pen and a clock.	2 points
Say, "No ifs, ands, or buts."	1 point
Three-step command:	3 points
Take a pencil in your right hand, put in your left hand, then put it on the floor.	
6. Read and obey the following:	
Close your eyes.	1 point
Write a sentence.	1 point
Copy design.	1 point
TOTAL	30 points

Fifteen percent of demented patients have a treatable and potentially reversible condition.

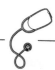

Minimum workup to exclude reversible causes of dementia:*
- CBC
- Electrolytes
- TFTs
- VDRL/RPR
- B_{12} and folate levels
- Brain CT or MRI

ETIOLOGY

The *most common* causes of dementia are:

1. Alzheimer's disease (50 to 60%)
2. Vascular dementia (10 to 20%)
3. Major depression ("pseudodementia")

DIFFERENTIAL DIAGNOSIS

Psychiatric
- Depression (pseudodementia)
- Delirium
- Schizophrenia
- Malingering

Organic

1. *Structural:* Benign forgetfulness of normal aging, Parkinson's disease, Huntington's disease, Down's syndrome, head trauma, brain tumor, normal pressure hydrocephalus, multiple sclerosis, subdural hematoma
2. *Metabolic:* Hypothyroidism, hypoxia, malnutrition (B_{12}, folate, or thiamine deficiency), Wilson's disease, lead toxicity
3. *Infectious:* Lyme disease, HIV dementia, Creutzfeldt–Jakob disease, neurosyphilis, meningitis, encephalitis

Drugs

- Alcohol (chronic and acute), phenothiazines, anticholinergics, sedatives

CLINICAL SCENARIOS OF DEMENTIA IN THE EXAM

Scenario	Think	Confirmatory/Diagnostic Tests
Dementia with stepwise increase in severity + focal neurological signs	Multi-infarct dementia	CT/MRI
Dementia + cogwheel rigidity + resting tremor	Lewy body dementia Parkinson's disease	Clinical
Dementia + ataxia + urinary incontinence + dilated cerebral ventricles	Normal pressure hydrocephalus	CT/MRI
Dementia + obesity + coarse hair + constipation + cold intolerance	Hypothyroidism	T_4, thyroid-stimulating hormone (TSH)
Dementia + diminished position and vibration sensation + megaloblasts on CBC	Vitamin B_{12} deficiency	Serum B_{12}
Dementia + tremor + abnormal liver function tests (LFTs) + Kayser–Fleischer rings	Wilson's disease	Ceruloplasmin
Dementia + diminished position and vibration sensation + **A**rgyll–**R**obertson **P**upils (**A**ccommodation **R**esponse **P**resent, response to light absent)	Neurosyphilis	Cerebrospinal fluid fluorescent treponemal antibody absorption test (CSF FTA-ABS) or CSF VDRL

▶ DELIRIUM

The hallmark of delirium is waxing/waning of consciousness. It can be caused by virtually any medical disorder, and there is a high mortality rate if untreated. It can last from days to weeks, and can also be chronic.

DSM-IV TREATMENT CRITERIA

The two types of delirium are:

1. *Quiet:* patient may seem depressed or exhibit symptoms similar to failure to thrive; an MMSE must be done to distinguish from depression and other diagnostic criteria
2. *Agitated:* obvious pulling out lines; may hallucinate

TREATMENT

- Rule out life-threatening causes
- Treat reversible causes, for example, hypothyroidism, electrolyte imbalance, urinary tract infections
- Antipsychotics first line: quetiapine (Seroquel) is excellent to use; also haloperidol PO/IM (do not use IV unless on cardiac monitor as it can cause torsades)

- Positive/negative use of benzodiazepines; can cause paradoxical disinhibition, respiratory depression, increased risk for falls
- 1:1 nursing for safety
- Frequently reorient patient.
- Avoid napping.
- Keep lights on, shades open during the day.
- In your orders, write "hold for sedation" after medication order so medications are not given when already sedated and calm.

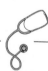

Differential for delirium: AEIOU TIPS
Alcohol
Electrolytes
Iatrogenic (anticholinergics, benzodiazepines, antiepileptics, blood pressure medicines, insulin, hypoglycemics, narcotics, steroids, H₂ receptor blockers, NSAIDs, antibiotics, antiparkinsonians)
Oxygen hypoxia (bleeding, central venous, pulmonary)
Uremia/hepatic encephalopathy

Trauma
Infection
Poisons
Seizures (post-ictal)

Differential between dementia and delirium is given in Table 8-2.

TABLE 8-2. Delirium Versus Dementia

Delirium	Dementia
Clouding of consciousness	Loss of memory/intellectual ability
Acute onset	*Insidious onset*
Lasts 3 days to 2 weeks	Lasts months to years
Orientation impaired	Orientation often impaired
Immediate/recent memory impaired	Recent and remote memory impaired
Visual hallucinations common	Hallucinations less common
Symptoms fluctuate, often worse at night	Symptoms stable throughout day
Usually reversible	15% reversible
Awareness reduced	Awareness clear
EEG changes (fast waves or generalized slowing)	*No EEG changes*

Alzheimer's Disease

Most common dementia (80% of all dementias)

EPIDEMIOLOGY

- Incidence: 5% of all people > 65; 15 to 25% of all people > 85
- More common in women than men
- Average life expectancy: 8 years after diagnosis
- Forty percent of patients have a family history of Alzheimer's.

CLINICAL MANIFESTATIONS

Hallmarks: Gradual progressive decline of cognitive functions, especially memory and language. Personality changes and mood swings are very common.

DIAGNOSIS AND DSM-IV CRITERIA

Memory impairment plus at least one of the following:
- **Aphasia**—disorder of language affecting speech *and* understanding
- **Apraxia**—inability to perform purposeful movements (e.g., copying a picture)
- **Agnosia**—inability to interpret sensations correctly (*visual* agnosia—inability to recognize a previously known object)
- **Diminished executive functioning**—problems with planning, organizing, and abstracting

APHASia is a disorder of language, speaking, and understanding **PHRASES**.
APRAXia: Can't do **PRAC**ticed movements like tying a shoe.
Ag**NOS**ia: Can't recognize things that were previously **KNOWN** (he used to know what a pencil was, but now he can't name it).

Personality/mood changes: Depression, anxiety, anger, and suspiciousness are common. Psychotic symptoms such as paranoia are common.

NEUROPHYSIOLOGY

Alzheimer's patients have decreased levels of acetylcholine (due to loss of noradrenergic neurons in the locus ceruleus of the brainstem) and of norepinephrine (due to preferential loss of cholinergic neurons in the basal nucleus of Meynert of the midbrain).

Pathological examination of the brain (at autopsy) is the only way to definitively diagnose Alzheimer's disease.

PATHOLOGY

Gross
- Diffuse atrophy with enlarged ventricles and flattened sulci

Microscopic
- *Senile plaques* composed of amyloid protein
- *Neurofibrillary tangles* derived from Tau proteins
- Neuronal and synaptic loss

Senile plaques and neurofibrillary tangles are not unique to Alzheimer's—they are also found in Down's syndrome and normal aging.

TREATMENT

- No cure or truly effective treatment
- Physical and emotional support, proper nutrition, exercise, and supervision
- NMDA receptor antagonists: memantine
- Cholinesterase inhibitors to help slow progression:
  - Tacrine (Cognex)
  - Donepezil (Aricept)
  - Rivastigmine (Exelon)
- Treatment of symptoms as necessary:
  - Low-dose, short-acting benzodiazepines for anxiety
  - Low-dose antipsychotics for agitation/psychosis (e.g., quetiapine)
  - Antidepressants for depression (if the patient fulfills criteria for major depression)

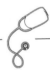

Cholinesterase inhibitors lead to a transient improvement in symptoms in only 25% of Alzheimer's patients.

Vascular Dementia

Caused by microvascular disease in the brain that produces multiple small infarcts. A substantial infarct burden must accumulate before dementia develops.

CLINICAL MANIFESTATIONS

Disease manifestations of vascular dementia are identical to Alzheimer's. **Memory impairment** and at least one of the following must be present:

1. **Aphasia**
2. **Apraxia**
3. **Agnosia**
4. Diminished executive functioning

Personality changes: Depression, anger, and suspiciousness are common. Psychotic symptoms such as paranoia are also common.

Classically, patients with vascular dementia have a **stepwise loss of function,** as the microinfarcts add up.

VASCULAR DEMENTIA VERSUS ALZHEIMER'S

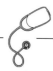

- Since vascular dementia is caused by small brain infarcts, patients also have focal neurological symptoms (such as hyperreflexia or paresthesias).
- Onset usually more abrupt than Alzheimer's
- Greater preservation of personality
- Can reduce risk by modifying risk factors (such as smoking, hypertension, and diabetes)

DIAGNOSIS

Can be diagnosed readily by MRI

TREATMENT

- No cure or truly effective treatment
- Physical and emotional support, proper nutrition, exercise, and supervision
- Treatment of symptoms as necessary

Mild cognitive impairment (MCI) is characterized by normal daily function but abnormal memory for age; most progress to Alzheimer's.

Pick's Disease/Frontotemporal Dementia (FTD)

A rare cause of slowly progressing dementia

CLINICAL MANIFESTATIONS

Hallmarks: Aphasia, apraxia, agnosia; difficult to distinguish from Alzheimer's clinically, but personality and behavioral changes are more prominent early in the disease

PATHOLOGY

- Atrophy of frontotemporal lobes
- **Pick bodies**—intraneuronal inclusion bodies (not necessary for diagnosis of FTD)

TREATMENT

- No effective treatment
- Physical, emotional, and nutritional support
- Treat emotional/behavioral symptoms as needed.

Huntington's Disease

Autosomal dominant genetic disorder that results in progressively disabling cognitive, physical, and psychological functioning, ultimately resulting in death after approximately 15 years

CLINICAL MANIFESTATIONS

- Onset: 35 to 50 years of age
- **Hallmarks:**
  - Progressive dementia
  - Bizarre **choreiform** movements (dancelike flailing of arms and legs)
  - Muscular hypertonicity
  - Depression and psychosis very common

Huntington's **D**isease
Hereditary
Autosomal **D**ominant

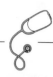

Choreiform movement =
Choreographed
(dancelike)

Pathology

Trinucleotide repeat on short arm of chromosome 4; primarily affects basal ganglia

Diagnosis

MRI shows caudate atrophy (and sometimes cortical atrophy). Genetic testing and MRI are diagnostic.

Treatment

There is no effective treatment available (supportive only).

Parkinson's Disease

Progressive disease with prominent neuronal loss in substantia nigra, which provides dopamine to the basal ganglia, causing physical and cognitive impairment. Approximately 30% of patients with Parkinson's disease develop dementia.

Clinical Manifestations

Characterized by:

1. Bradykinesia
2. Cogwheel rigidity
3. Resting tremor—"pill-rolling" tremor most common
4. Masklike facial expression
5. Shuffling gait
6. Dysarthria (abnormal speech)

Fifty percent of patients will suffer from depression. Dementia symptoms resemble Alzheimer's type. Muhammad Ali (advanced) and Michael J. Fox (early) both suffer from Parkinson's.

Etiology

- Idiopathic (most common)
- Traumatic (e.g., Muhammad Ali)
- Drug- or toxin-induced
- Encephalitic (as in the book/movie *Awakenings*)
- Familial (rare)

Pathology and Pathophysiology

Loss of cells in the substantia nigra of the basal ganglia, which leads to a decrease in dopamine and loss of the dopaminergic tracts

Treatment

Pharmacologic
- Levodopa—degraded to dopamine by dopadecarboxylase
- Carbidopa—peripheral dopadecarboxylase inhibitor prevents levodopa from being converted to dopamine before it reaches the brain.
- Amantadine—mechanism unknown
- Anticholinergics—help relieve tremor
- Dopamine agonists (bromocriptine, etc.)
- Monoamine oxidase (MAO)-B inhibitors (selegiline)—inhibit breakdown of dopamine

Cortical dementias include Alzheimer's, Pick's, and CJD and are marked by decline in intellectual functioning. *Subcortical* dementias include Huntington's, Parkinson's, NPH, and multi-infarct dementia and have more prominent affective and movement symptoms.

Levodopa crosses the blood–brain barrier (BBB). Carbidopa does not. Carbidopa prevents conversion of levodopa to dopamine in the periphery. Once levodopa crosses BBB, it is free to be converted to dopamine.

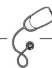

Amanta**din**e **eman**cipates dopam**ine**.

Surgical

Thalamotomy or pallidotomy may be performed if no longer responsive to pharmacotherapy.

Creutzfeldt–Jakob Disease (CJD)

A rapidly progressive, degenerative disease of the central nervous system (CNS) caused by a *prion*. CJD may be inherited, sporadic, or acquired. A small percentage of patients have become infected through corneal transplants.

CLINICAL MANIFESTATIONS

PRions are **PR**oteinaceous infectious particles that are normally expressed by healthy neurons of the brain. Accumulations of *abnormal forms* of prions are responsible for disease.

Hallmarks: Rapidly progressive dementia 6 to 12 months after onset of symptoms. More than 90% of patients have myoclonus (sudden spasms of muscles). Extrapyramidal signs, ataxia, and lower motor neuron signs are also common. There is a long latency period between exposure and disease onset.

Other prion diseases:
- Kuru
- Gerstmann–Straussler syndrome
- Fatal familial insomnia
- Bovine spongiform encephalopathy ("mad cow disease")

PATHOLOGY

Spongiform changes of cerebral cortex, neuronal loss, and hypertrophy of glial cells

DIAGNOSIS

EEG in CJD: Periodic sharp waves/spikes
Pathology of CJD: Spongiform changes

Definitive—pathological demonstration of spongiform changes of brain tissue
Probable—the presence of both rapidly progressive dementia and periodic generalized sharp waves on electroencephalogram (EEG) *plus* at least two of the following clinical features:
- Myoclonus
- Cortical blindness
- Ataxia, pyramidal signs, or extrapyramidal signs
- Muscle atrophy
- Mutism

TREATMENT AND COURSE

No treatment; relentless course, progressing to death usually within a year

Normal Pressure Hydrocephalus (NPH)

NPH is a reversible cause of dementia. Patients have enlarged ventricles with increased CSF pressure. The etiology is either idiopathic or secondary to obstruction of CSF reabsorption sites due to trauma, infection, or hemorrhage.

CLINICAL MANIFESTATIONS

Clinical triad:

1. Gait disturbance (often appears first)
2. Urinary incontinence
3. Dementia (mild, insidious onset)

TREATMENT

Relieve increased pressure with shunt. Of the clinical triad, the dementia is least likely to improve.

▶ DELIRIUM

Delirium is an acute disorder of cognition related to impairment of cerebral metabolism. Unlike demented patients, delirious patients have a **rapid onset** of symptoms, periods of **altered levels of consciousness,** and **potential reversal** of symptoms with treatment of the underlying cause.

Delirious patients appear confused and have a fluctuating course with **lucid intervals.** They may be either stuporous or agitated, and perceptual disturbances (e.g., **hallucinations**) are common. Patients are often anxious, incoherent, and unable to sleep normally.

ETIOLOGY

Common causes of delirium include:
- CNS injury or disease
- Systemic illness
- Drug abuse/withdrawal
- Hypoxia

Additional causes of delirium include:
- Fever
- Sensory deprivation
- Medications (anticholinergics, steroids, antipsychotics, antihypertensives, insulin, etc.)
- Postop
- Electrolyte imbalances

DIFFERENTIAL DIAGNOSIS

Dementia, fluent aphasia (Wernicke's), acute amnestic syndrome, psychosis, depression, malingering

TREATMENT

- First and foremost: Treat the underlying cause!
- Provide physical and sensory support.
- Treat drug withdrawal.
- Treat symptoms of psychosis (low-dose antipsychotic) and insomnia (sedative-hypnotic).

Clinical Scenarios of Delirium in the Exam

Since a delirium is not a primary pathophysiological process but secondary to another, it is helpful to consider various scenarios (like the following) and determine the proper diagnostic approach for the patient.

Delirium is common in intensive care unit setting/acute medical illness and has increased incidence in children and elderly.

Causes of delirium: I'M DELIRIOUS
Impaired delivery (of brain substrates, such as vascular insufficiency due to stroke)
Metabolic

Drugs
Endocrinopathy
Liver disease
Infrastructure (structural disease of cortical neurons)
Renal failure
Infection
Oxygen
Urinary tract infection
Sensory deprivation

Scenario	Think	Confirmatory Diagnostic Tests
Delirium + hemiparesis or other focal neurological signs and symptoms	Cerebrovascular accident (CVA) or mass lesion	Brain CT/MRI
Delirium + elevated blood pressure + papilledema	Hypertensive encephalopathy	Brain CT/MRI
Delirium + dilated pupils + tachycardia	Drug intoxication	Urine toxicology screen
Delirium + fever + nuchal rigidity + photophobia	**Meningitis**	Lumbar puncture
Delirium + tachycardia + tremor + thyromegaly	Thyrotoxicosis	T_4, TSH

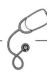

Treating a delirious patient is often a **FEUD:**
Fluids/Nutrition
Environment
Underlying cause
Drug withdrawal

Avoid using benzodiazepines in delirious patients, as they will often exacerbate the delirium.

► **AMNESTIC DISORDERS**

Amnestic disorders cause impairment of memory without other cognitive problems or altered consciousness. They always occur secondary to an underlying *medical* condition. (See chapter on Dissociative Disorders for discussion of amnestic syndromes caused by *psychiatric* disorders.)

ETIOLOGY

Causes of amnestic disorders include:
- Hypoglycemia
- Systemic illness (such as thiamine deficiency)
- Hypoxia
- Head trauma
- Brain tumor
- CVA
- Seizures
- Multiple sclerosis
- Herpes simplex encephalitis
- Substance use (alcohol, benzodiazepines, medications)

COURSE AND PROGNOSIS

Variable depending on underlying medical cause:
Usually transient with full recovery: Seizures, medication-induced
Possibly permanent: Hypoxia, head trauma, herpes simplex encephalitis, CVA

TREATMENT

- Treatment of underlying cause
- Supportive psychotherapy if needed (to help patients accept their limits and understand their course of recovery)

Geriatric Psychiatry

▶ INTRODUCTION

The geriatric population of the United States is growing faster than any other segment. Though the elderly are susceptible to the same Axis I disorders as younger adults, certain diagnoses are more prevalent in this population, such as cognitive disorders and major depression. Also, illnesses often have different clinical presentations in the elderly and may require unique treatments.

Approach to the Geriatric Patient

Geriatric patients should undergo the same psychiatric assessment as younger adults, including the mental status exam. In patients who suffer from cognitive disorders, family members or caretakers may need to be interviewed to obtain collateral information. A careful history of current medications should be taken, as drugs often produce adverse behavioral, cognitive, and psychiatric symptoms in the elderly, and elderly individuals may be taking multiple medications at the same time.

Normal Aging

Factors associated with normal aging include:
- Decreased muscle mass/increased fat
- Decreased brain weight/enlarged ventricles and sulci
- Impaired vision and hearing
- Minor forgetfulness (called *benign senescent forgetfulness*)

Stages of Dying

Normal emotional responses when facing death or loss of a body part include:
- Denial
- Anger (blaming others for illness)
- Bargaining ("I'll never smoke or drink again if my cancer is cured.")
- Depression
- Acceptance

Stages of dying may be experienced in any order and may occur simultaneously. A person of any age who is dealing with loss or death experiences these same stages.

Work up an elderly patient for major depression when he or she presents with memory loss.

▶ MAJOR DEPRESSION

Major depression is a common mental disorder in the geriatric population, and the elderly are twice as likely to commit suicide as the general population. Depressive symptoms are present in 15% of nursing home residents.

Symptoms of major depression in the elderly often include problems with memory and cognitive functioning; because this clinical picture may be mistaken for dementia, it is termed *pseudodementia*.

▶ PSEUDODEMENTIA

Pseudodementia is the presence of apparent cognitive deficits in patients with major depression. Patients may appear demented; however, their symptoms are only secondary to their underlying depression. It can be difficult to differentiate the two.

PSEUDODEMENTIA VERSUS DEMENTIA

See Table 9-1.

CLINICAL MANIFESTATIONS

Demented patients are more likely to confabulate when they do not know an answer, whereas depressed patients will just say they do not know: when pressed for an answer, depressed patients will often give the correct one.

Important clinical note: Depressed elderly patients often present with physical symptoms, such as stomach pain, or with memory loss associated with pseudodementia. *Always investigate a possible diagnosis of major depression when an elderly person presents with nonspecific complaints such as these.*

Depressive symptoms include:
- Sleep disturbances (early morning awakenings)
- Decreased appetite and weight loss
- Feelings of worthlessness and suicidal ideation
- Lack of energy and diminished interest in activities

TABLE 9-1. Dementia Versus Pseudodementia (Depression)

Dementia	Pseudodementia (Depression)
Onset is insidious	Onset is more acute
Patient delights in accomplishments	Patient emphasizes failures
Sundowning common (increased confusion at night)	Sundowning uncommon
Will guess at answers (confabulate)	Often answers "Don't know"
Patient unaware of problems	Patient is aware of problems

TREATMENT

- Supportive psychotherapy
- Psychodynamic psychotherapy if indicated
- Low-dose antidepressant medication (selective serotonin reuptake inhibitors [SSRIs] have the fewest side effects and are usually preferable to tricyclics or monoamine oxidase [MAO] inhibitors).
- Electroconvulsive therapy (ECT) may be used in place of medication (safe and effective in the elderly).
- Mirtazapine can potentially increase appetite; is also sedating, and therefore good for insomnia.
- Methylphenidate can be used at low doses as an adjunct to antidepressants for patients with psychomotor retardation; however, do not give in late afternoon or evening as it can cause insomnia.

The elderly are very sensitive to side effects of antidepressant medications, particularly anticholinergics.

▶ BEREAVEMENT

The elderly are more likely to experience losses of loved ones or friends. It is important to be able to distinguish normal grief reactions from pathological ones (depression).

Normal grief may involve:
- Feelings of guilt and sadness
- Mild sleep disturbance and weight loss
- Illusions (briefly seeing the deceased person or hearing his or her voice—these tend to be culturally related, i.e., in some cultures this is the norm, not the exception)
- Attempts to resume daily activities/work
- Symptoms that resolve within 1 year (worst symptoms within 2 months)

Abnormal grief (major depression) may involve:
- Feelings of severe guilt and worthlessness
- Significant sleep disturbance and weight loss
- Hallucinations or delusions
- No attempt to resume activities
- Suicidal ideation
- Symptoms persist more than 1 year (worst symptoms more than 2 months).

▶ SLEEP DISTURBANCES

The incidence of sleep disorders increases with aging. Elderly people often report difficulty sleeping, daytime drowsiness, and daytime napping. The causes of sleep disturbances may include general medical conditions, environment, and medications, as well as normal changes associated with aging.

CHANGES IN SLEEP STRUCTURE

The structure of sleep changes normally with aging:
- *Rapid eye movement (REM) sleep:* Increased number of REM episodes throughout the night. These episodes are redistributed throughout the sleep cycle and are shorter than normal. Total amount of REM sleep remains about the same as with younger adults.

■ *Non-REM sleep:* Increased amount of stage 1 and 2 sleep with a decrease in stage 3 and 4 sleep (deep sleep); increased awakening after sleep onset

DIFFERENTIAL DIAGNOSIS

Causes of sleep disorders in the elderly include:
- Primary sleep disorder (most common is *primary insomnia;* others include nocturnal myoclonus, restless leg syndrome, and sleep apnea)
- Other mental disorders
- General medical conditions
- Social/environmental factors (alcohol consumption, lack of daily structure, etc.)

TREATMENT

Sedative-hypnotic drugs are more likely to cause side effects when used by the elderly, including memory impairment, ataxia, paradoxical excitement, and rebound insomnia. Therefore, other approaches should be tried first, including alcohol cessation, increased structure of daily routine, elimination of daytime naps, and treatment of underlying medical conditions that may be exacerbating sleep problems. If sedative-hypnotics must be prescribed, medications such as hydroxyzine (Vistaril) or zolpidem (Ambien) are safer than the more sedating benzodiazepines.

▶ ELDER ABUSE

INCIDENCE

- Ten percent of all people > 65 years old; underreported by victims
- Perpetrator is usually a caregiver who lives with the victim.

TYPES

Physical abuse, sexual abuse, psychological abuse (threats, insults, etc.), neglect (withholding of care), and exploitation (misuse of finances)

▶ CARE FOR THE ELDERLY

Restraints

Restraints are often overused in nursing homes and hospitals. Patients who are restrained suffer both physically and psychologically. Always try alternatives such as closer monitoring or tilted chairs.

Medications

Many older people are on multiple medications. They suffer from more side effects because of decreased lean body mass and impaired liver and kidney function. When confronted with a new symptom in an elderly patient on multiple medications, always try to remove a medication before adding one.

Nursing Homes

Provide care and rehabilitation for chronically ill and impaired patients as well as for patients who are in need of short-term care before returning to their prior living arrangements. Approximately half the patients stay on permanently, and half are discharged after only a few months.

Old-Age Homes

Institutions in which the elderly can live for the rest of their lives, with no attempt to rehabilitate.

HIGH-YIELD FACTS

Geriatric Psychiatry

Psychiatric Disorders in Children

In child psychiatry, it is important to consult multiple sources when gathering information:

- **The child**—young children usually report information in *concrete terms* but give accurate details about their *emotional states*.
- **Parents**—generally more reliable for information about the child's *conduct*, school performance, or problems with the law. Parents should be asked about the child's *developmental history* and about issues with other family members (medical or psychiatric conditions, problems in family functioning, etc.).
- **Teachers**—may reveal important collateral information about the child's conduct, academic performance, and peer relationships
- **Child welfare/juvenile justice**—if applicable

Other Methods of Gathering Information

- **Play, stories, drawing**—help to assess conceptualization, internal states, experiences, and the like
- **Kaufman Assessment Battery for Children (K-ABC)**—intelligence test for ages 2½ to 12
- **Weschler Intelligence Scale for Children–Revised (WISC-R)**—determines intelligence quotient (IQ) for ages 6 to 16
- **Peabody Individual Achievement Test (PIAT)**—tests academic achievement

Mental retardation is defined by the DSM-IV as:

- Significantly subaverage intellectual functioning with an IQ of 70 or below
- Deficits in adaptive skills appropriate for the age group
- Onset must be before the age of 18.

EPIDEMIOLOGY

- Affects 2.5% of the population
- Approximately 85% of mentally retarded are mild cases
- Males affected twice as often as females

SUBCLASSIFICATIONS

Type of MR	Definition	% of MR
Profound	IQ < 25	1 to 2% of MR
Severe	IQ 25–40	3 to 4% of MR
Moderate	IQ 40–50	10% of MR
Mild	IQ 50–70	80% of MR

CAUSES

Most MR has no identifiable cause.

Genetic
- **Down's syndrome**—trisomy 21 (1/700 live births)
- **Fragile X syndrome**—second most common cause of retardation; involves mutation of X chromosome; affects males more than females
- Many others

Prenatal: Infection and Toxins (TORCH)
- **T**oxoplasmosis
- **O**ther (syphilis, AIDS, alcohol/illicit drugs)
- **R**ubella (German measles)
- **C**ytomegalovirus (CMV)
- **H**erpes simplex

Perinatal
- Anoxia
- Prematurity
- Birth trauma

Postnatal
- Hypothyroidism
- Malnutrition
- Toxin exposure
- Trauma

Always rule out a hearing or visual deficit in the workup before diagnosing learning disorders.

▶ LEARNING DISORDERS

Learning disorders are defined by the DSM-IV as achievement in reading, mathematics, or written expression that is significantly lower than expected for chronological age, level of education, and level of intelligence. Learning disorders affect academic achievement or daily activities and cannot be explained by sensory deficits, poor teaching, or cultural factors. They are often due to deficits in cognitive processing (abnormal attention, memory, visual perception, etc.).

Types of learning disorders include:

- Reading disorder
- Mathematics disorder
- Disorder of written expression
- Learning disorder not otherwise specified (NOS)

EPIDEMIOLOGY

Reading Disorder
- 4% of school-age children
- Boys affected 3 to 4 times as often as girls

Mathematics Disorder
- 5% of school-age children
- May be more common in girls

Disorder of Written Expression
- Affects 3 to 10% of school-age children
- Male-to-female ratio unknown

ETIOLOGY

Learning disorders may be caused by genetic factors, abnormal development, perinatal injury, and neurological or medical conditions.

TREATMENT

Remedial education tailored to the child's specific needs

▶ DISRUPTIVE BEHAVIORAL DISORDERS

Disruptive behavioral disorders include conduct disorder and oppositional defiant disorder.

Conduct Disorder

DIAGNOSIS AND DSM-IV CRITERIA

A pattern of behavior that involves violation of the basic rights of others or of social norms and rules, with at least three acts within the following categories during the past year:

1. Aggression toward people and animals
2. Destruction of property
3. Deceitfulness
4. Serious violations of rules

EPIDEMIOLOGY

- Prevalence: 6 to 16% in boys, 2 to 9% in girls
- Etiology involves genetic and psychosocial factors.
- Up to 40% risk of developing antisocial personality disorder in adulthood
- Increased incidence of comorbid attention deficit hyperactivity disorder and learning disorders
- Increased incidence of comorbid mood disorders, substance abuse, and criminal behavior in adulthood

A 9-year-old boy's mother has been called to school because her son has been hitting other children and stealing their pens. His mother reveals that he often pokes the cat they have at home with sharp objects. *Think: Conduct disorder.*

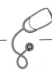

Conduct disorder is the most common diagnosis in outpatient child psychiatry clinics.

TREATMENT

A multimodal treatment approach is most effective. It is important to structure the child's environment with firm rules that are consistently enforced. Individual psychotherapy that focuses on behavior modification and problem-solving skills is often useful. Adjunctive pharmacotherapy may be helpful, including antipsychotics or lithium for aggression and selective serotonin reuptake inhibitors (SSRIs) for impulsivity, irritability, and mood lability.

Oppositional Defiant Disorder (ODD)

DIAGNOSIS AND DSM-IV CRITERIA

At least 6 months of negativistic, hostile, and defiant behavior during which at least four of the following have been present:

1. Frequent loss of temper
2. Arguments with adults
3. Defying adults' rules
4. Deliberately annoying people
5. Easily annoyed
6. Anger and resentment
7. Spiteful
8. Blaming others for mistakes or misbehaviors

EPIDEMIOLOGY

- Prevalence: 16 to 22% in children > age 6
- Usually begins by age 8
- Onset before puberty more common in boys; onset after puberty equal in boys and girls
- Increased incidence of comorbid substance abuse, mood disorders, and attention deficit hyperactivity disorder
- Remits in 25% of children; may progress to conduct disorder

TREATMENT

Treatment should involve individual psychotherapy that focuses on behavior modification and problem-solving skills as well as parenting skills training.

▶ ATTENTION DEFICIT HYPERACTIVITY DISORDER (ADHD)

There are three subcategories of ADHD: Predominantly inattentive type, predominantly hyperactive–impulsive type, and combined type.

DIAGNOSIS AND DSM-IV CRITERIA

1. At least six symptoms involving inattentiveness, hyperactivity, or both that have persisted for at least 6 months:
   - **Inattention**—problems listening, concentrating, paying attention to details, or organizing tasks; easily distracted, often forgetful
   - **Hyperactivity–impulsivity**—blurting out, interrupting, fidgeting, leaving seat, talking excessively, and so on
2. Onset before age 7
3. Behavior inconsistent with age and development

Unlike conduct disorder, ODD does not involve violation of the basic rights of others.

A 9-year-old boy's mother has been called to school because her son is defiant toward the teachers and does not comply in any class activities. His behavior is appropriate toward his classmates. *Think: Oppositional defiant disorder (ODD).*

Two thirds of children with ADHD also have conduct disorder or ODD.

A 9-year-old boy's mother has been called to school because her son has not been doing his homework. He claims he did not know about the assignments. He interrupts other kids during class and according to the teacher, "never sits still." *Think: Attention deficit hyperactivity disorder (ADHD).*

EPIDEMIOLOGY

- 3 to 5% prevalence in school-age children
- Three to five times more common in boys
- Increased incidence of comorbid mood disorders, personality disorders, conduct disorder, and ODD
- Most cases remit in adolescence; 20% of patients have symptoms into adulthood.

ETIOLOGY

The etiology of ADHD is multifactorial, including:

- Genetic factors (higher incidence in monozygotic twins than dizygotic)
- Prenatal trauma/toxin exposure (e.g., fetal alcohol syndrome, lead poisoning, etc.)
- Neurochemical factors (dysregulation of peripheral and central noradrenergic systems)
- Neurophysiological factors (can be demonstrated in certain patients with abnormal electroencephalogram [EEG] patterns or positron-emission tomography scans)
- Psychosocial factors (emotional deprivation, etc.)

Depression in children and adolescents may be manifested primarily as irritableness instead of dysphoria. Otherwise, the criteria for the depressive disorders are the same as for adults.

TREATMENT

1. Pharmacotherapy:
   - CNS stimulants—methylphenidate (Ritalin) is first-line therapy, dextroamphetamine (Dexedrine), and pemoline (Cylert)
   - SSRIs/tricyclic antidepressants (TCAs)—adjunctive therapy
2. Individual psychotherapy—with focus on behavior modification techniques
3. Parental counseling (education and parenting skills training)
4. Group therapy—to help patient improve social skills, self-esteem, etc.

Ritalin is considered first-line therapy in ADHD; significant improvement is seen in 75% of patients.

▶ PERVASIVE DEVELOPMENTAL DISORDERS (PDD)

Pervasive developmental disorders are a group of conditions that involve problems with social skills, language, and behaviors. Impairment is noticeable at an early age of life and involves multiple areas of development.

Examples of PDD include:

- Autistic disorder
- Asperger's disorder
- Rett's disorder
- Childhood disintegrative disorder

Autistic Disorder

DIAGNOSIS AND DSM-IV CRITERIA

To diagnose autism, at least six symptoms from the following categories must be present:

1. **Problems with social interaction** (at least two):
   - Impairment in nonverbal behaviors (facial expression, gestures, etc.)
   - Failure to develop peer relationships

A 3-year-old boy is brought in by his parents because they think he is deaf. According to the parents, he shows no interest in them or anyone around him and only speaks when spoken to directly. He often takes his toys and lines them up in a straight line. His hearing tests are normal. *Think: Autism.*

- Failure to seek sharing of interests or enjoyment with others
- Lack of social/emotional reciprocity
2. **Impairments in communication** (at least one)
   - Lack of or delayed speech
   - Repetitive use of language
   - Lack of varied, spontaneous play, and so on
3. **Repetitive and stereotyped patterns of behavior and activities** (at least one)
   - Inflexible rituals
   - Preoccupation with parts of objects, and so on

EPIDEMIOLOGY

- Incidence of 0.02 to 0.05% in children under age 12
- Boys have 3 to 5 times higher incidence than girls
- Some familial inheritance
- Significant association with fragile X syndrome, tuberous sclerosis, mental retardation, and seizures
- Autism may be apparent at an early age due to delayed developmental milestones (social smile, facial expression, etc.). It almost always begins before age 3.
- Seventy percent of patients with autism are mentally retarded (IQ < 70). Only 1 to 2% can function completely independently as adults.

ETIOLOGY

The etiology of autism is multifactorial, including:
- Prenatal neurological insults (from infections, drugs, etc.)
- Genetic factors (36% concordance rate in monozygotic twins)
- Immunological and biochemical factors

TREATMENT

There is no cure for autism, but various treatments are used to help manage symptoms and improve social skills:
- Remedial education
- Behavioral therapy
- Neuroleptics (to help control aggression, hyperactivity, and mood lability)
- SSRIs (adjunctive therapy to help control stereotyped and repetitive behaviors)
- Some children benefit from stimulants.

Asperger's Disorder

DIAGNOSIS AND DSM-IV CRITERIA

Unlike autistic disorder, children with Asperger's disorder have normal language and cognitive development.

1. **Impaired social interaction (at least two):**
   - Failure to develop peer relationships
   - Impaired use of nonverbal behaviors (facial expression, gestures, etc.)
   - Lack of seeking to share enjoyment or interests with others
   - Lack of social/emotional reciprocity
2. **Restricted or stereotyped behaviors, interests, or activities** (inflexible routines, repetitive movements, preoccupations, etc.)

EPIDEMIOLOGY

- Incidence unknown
- Boys > girls

ETIOLOGY

Unknown etiology; may involve genetic, infectious, or perinatal factors

TREATMENT

Supportive treatment; similar to autistic disorder (see above). Social skills training and behavioral modification techniques may be useful.

Rett's Disorder

Rett's disorder is characterized by:

1. Normal prenatal and perinatal development
2. Normal psychomotor development during the first 5 months after birth
3. Normal head circumference at birth, but decreasing rate of head growth between the ages of 5 and 48 months
4. Loss of previously learned purposeful hand skills between ages 5 and 30 months, followed by development of stereotyped hand movements (such as hand wringing, hand washing, etc.)
5. Early loss of social interaction, usually followed by subsequent improvement
6. Problems with gait or trunk movements
7. Severely impaired language and psychomotor development
8. Seizures
9. Cyanotic spells

Rett's disorder is seen only in girls; early development appears normal, but diminished head circumference and stereotyped hand movements eventually ensue. Cognitive development never progresses beyond that of the first year of life.

EPIDEMIOLOGY

- Onset between age 5 and 48 months
- Seen in girls predominantly
- Boys have variable phenotype, characterized predominantly by developmental delay; many die *in utero*
- Rare
- Genetic testing is available

ETIOLOGY

MECP2 gene mutation on X chromosome.

TREATMENT

Supportive

Childhood Disintegrative Disorder

DIAGNOSIS AND DSM-IV CRITERIA

1. Normal development in the first 2 years of life
2. Loss of previously acquired skills in at least two of the following areas:
   - Language
   - Social skills

- Bowel or bladder control
- Play
- Motor skills

3. At least two of the following:
   - Impaired social interaction
   - Impaired use of language
   - Restricted, repetitive, and stereotyped behaviors and interests

EPIDEMIOLOGY

- Onset age 2 to 10
- Four to eight times higher incidence in boys than girls
- Rare

ETIOLOGY

Unknown

TREATMENT

Supportive (similar to that of autistic disorder)

Tics in Tourette's may be consciously suppressed for brief periods of time.

▶ TOURETTE'S DISORDER AND TIC DISORDERS

Tics are involuntary movements or vocalizations. Tourette's disorder is the most severe tic disorder and is characterized by multiple daily motor or vocal tics with onset before age 18. Vocal tics may first appear many years after the motor tics. The most common **motor tics** involve the face and head, such as blinking of the eyes. Examples of **vocal tics** include:

- *Coprolalia*—repetitive speaking of obscene words (uncommon in children)
- *Echolalia*—exact repetition of words

Both motor and vocal tics must be present to diagnose Tourette's disorder. The presence of exclusive motor or vocal tics suggests a diagnosis of motor tic disorder or vocal tic disorder.

DIAGNOSIS AND DSM-IV CRITERIA

- Multiple motor and vocal tics (both must be present)
- Tics occur many times a day, almost every day for > 1 year (no tic-free period > 3 months)
- Onset prior to age 18
- Distress or impairment in social/occupational functioning

EPIDEMIOLOGY

- Occurs in 0.05% of children
- Three times more common in boys than girls
- Onset usually between ages 7 and 8
- High co-morbidity with obsessive–compulsive disorder and ADHD

ETIOLOGY

A 13-year-old boy has had uncontrollable blinking tics since he was 9 years old. Lately, he has noticed that he often involuntarily makes a barking noise that is very embarrassing.
Think: Tourette's disorder.

- Genetic factors—50% concordance rate in monozygotic versus 8% in dizygotic twins
- Neurochemical factors—impaired regulation of **dopamine** in the caudate nucleus (and possibly impaired regulation of endogenous opiates and the noradrenergic system)

TREATMENT

- Pharmacotherapy—haloperidol or pimozide (dopamine receptor antagonists)
- Supportive psychotherapy

▶ ELIMINATION DISORDERS

Enuresis

Urinary continence is normally established before age 4. Enuresis is the involuntary voiding of urine (bedwetting). Rule out medical conditions (urethritis, diabetes, seizures).

Primary—child never established urinary continence.
Secondary—manifestation occurs after a period of urinary continence, most commonly between ages 5 and 8.
Diurnal—includes daytime episodes
Nocturnal—includes nighttime episodes

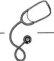

The great majority of cases of enuresis spontaneously remit by age 7.

DIAGNOSIS AND DSM-IV CRITERIA

- Involuntary voiding after age 5
- Occurs at least twice a week for 3 months or with marked impairment

EPIDEMIOLOGY

Occurs in 7% of of 5-year-olds; prevalence decreases with age.

ETIOLOGY

- Genetic predisposition
- Small bladder or low nocturnal levels of antidiuretic hormone
- Psychological stress

TREATMENT

- Behavior modification (such as buzzer that wakes child up when sensor detects wetness)
- Pharmacotherapy—antidiuretics (DDAVP) or TCAs (such as imipramine).

Encopresis

Bowel control is normally achieved by the age of 4. Bowel incontinence can result in rejection by peers and impairment of social development. One must rule out conditions such as metabolic abnormalities (such as hypothyroidism), lower gastrointestinal problems (anal fissure, inflammatory bowel disease), and dietary factors.

DIAGNOSIS AND DSM-IV CRITERIA

- Involuntary or intentional passage of feces in inappropriate places
- Must be at least 4 years of age
- Has occurred at least once a month for 3 months

EPIDEMIOLOGY

- Occurs in 1% of 5-year-old children
- Incidence decreases with age
- Associated with other psychiatric conditions, such as conduct disorder and ADHD

ETIOLOGY

- Psychosocial stressors
- Lack of sphincter control
- Constipation with overflow incontinence

TREATMENT

- Psychotherapy, family therapy, and behavioral therapy
- Stool softeners (if etiology is constipation)

► **OTHER CHILDHOOD DISORDERS**

Selective Mutism

Selective mutism is a rare condition that occurs more commonly in girls than in boys. It is characterized by not speaking in certain situations (such as in school). Onset is usually around age 5 or 6, and it may be preceded by a stressful life event. Treatment involves supportive psychotherapy, behavior therapy, and family therapy.

Separation Anxiety Disorder

Separation anxiety disorder involves excessive fear of leaving one's parents or other major attachment figures. Children with this disorder may refuse to go to school or to sleep alone. They may complain of physical symptoms in order to avoid having to go to school. When forced to separate, they become extremely distressed and may worry excessively about losing their parents forever.

Separation anxiety disorder affects up to 4% of school-age children and occurs equally in boys and girls. Onset is usually around age 7 and may be preceded by a stressful life event. Parents are often afflicted with anxiety disorders and may express excessive concern about their children. Treatment involves family therapy, supportive psychotherapy, and low-dose antidepressants.

Child Abuse

Child abuse includes physical abuse, emotional abuse, sexual abuse, and neglect. Doctors are legally required to report all cases of suspected child abuse to appropriate social service agencies. In cases of suspected abuse, children may be admitted to the hospital without parental consent in order to protect them.

Adults who were abused as children have an increased risk of developing anxiety disorders, depressive disorders, dissociative disorders, substance abuse disorders, and posttraumatic stress disorder. They also have an increased risk of subsequently abusing their own children.

SEXUAL ABUSE

- Child sexual abuse most often involves a male who knows the child. The existence of true pedophilia in the abuser is rare.
- Children are most commonly sexually abused between the ages of 9 and 12.
- Twenty-five percent of women and 12% of men report having been sexually abused as children.

Evidence of sexual abuse in a child:
- Sexually transmitted diseases
- Anal or genital trauma
- Knowledge about specific sexual acts (inappropriate for age)
- Initiation of sexual activity with others
- Sexual play with dolls (inappropriate for age)

Psychiatric Disorders in Children

Dissociative Disorders

▶ DEFINITION

Dissociative disorders are defined by a loss of memory, identity, or sense of self (one's sense of self is the normal integration of one's thoughts, behaviors, perceptions, feelings, and memory into a unique identity). Amnesia and feelings of detachment often arise suddenly and may be temporary in duration. Examples of dissociative disorders include:

- Dissociative amnesia
- Dissociative fugue
- Dissociative identity disorder (multiple personality disorder)
- Depersonalization disorder

Unlike the amnesia present in amnestic disorders, symptoms of dissociative disorders are never due to an underlying medical condition or substance use. Instead, their onset is related to a stressful life event or personal problem. Many patients with dissociative disorders have a history of trauma or abuse during childhood. Amnesia secondary to *medical* conditions is found in the "amnestic disorders" (discussed in the cognitive disorders chapter).

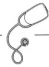

The phenomenon of dissociation ranges from nonpathologic, such as the state of mind entered during hypnosis, to extremely pathological, as seen in multiple personality disorder.

▶ DISSOCIATIVE AMNESIA

Amnesia is a prominent symptom in all of the dissociative disorders except depersonalization disorder. However, the diagnosis of dissociative amnesia requires that amnesia be the only dissociative symptom present. Patients with this disorder are usually aware that they are having difficulty remembering but are not very troubled by it.

DIAGNOSIS AND DSM-IV CRITERIA

- At least one episode of inability to recall important personal information, usually involving a traumatic or stressful event
- The amnesia cannot be explained by ordinary forgetfulness.
- Symptoms cause significant distress or impairment in daily functioning and cannot be explained by another disorder, medical condition, or substance use.

Patients are often unable to recall their name or other important information but will remember obscure details. This is opposite to the type of memory loss usually found in dementia.

A 28-year-old woman is unable to recall any events of her rape in which she was hospitalized for 2 months. *Think: Dissociative amnesia.*

Abreaction is the strong reaction patients often get when retrieving traumatic memories.

Dissociative **Fug**ue — **Fug**itives take off and form new identities.

Unlike dissociative amnesia, patients with dissociative fugue are not aware that they have forgotten anything.

EPIDEMIOLOGY

- Most common dissociative disorder
- More common in women than men
- More common in younger adults than older
- Increased incidence of comorbid major depression and anxiety disorders

COURSE AND PROGNOSIS

Many patients abruptly return to normal after minutes or days. Recurrences are uncommon.

TREATMENT

It is important to help patients retrieve their lost memories in order to prevent future recurrences. Hypnosis or administration of sodium amobarbital or lorazepam during the interview may be useful to help patients talk more freely. Subsequent psychotherapy is then recommended. Ativan is used more frequently than sodium amobarbital, as it is safer and better tolerated (lower risk of respiratory depression).

▶ DISSOCIATIVE FUGUE

Dissociative fugue is characterized by sudden, unexpected travel away from home, accompanied by the inability to recall parts of one's past or identity. Patients often assume an entirely new identity and occupation after arriving in the new location. They are *unaware* of their amnesia and new identity, and they never recall the period of the fugue.

DIAGNOSIS AND DSM-IV CRITERIA

- Sudden, unexpected travel away from home or work plus inability to recall one's past
- Confusion about personal identity or assumption of new identity
- Not due to dissociative identity disorder or the physiological effects of a substance or medical disorder
- Symptoms cause impairment in social or occupational functioning.

EPIDEMIOLOGY

- Rare
- Predisposing factors include heavy use of alcohol, major depression, history of head trauma, and epilepsy
- Onset associated with stressful life event (dissociative fugue is often viewed as a response to a life stressor or personal conflict)

COURSE AND PROGNOSIS

The fugue usually lasts a few hours to several days but may last longer. After the episode, the patient will assume his or her old identity without ever remembering the time of the fugue.

TREATMENT

Similar to that of dissociative amnesia (see above)

▶ DISSOCIATIVE IDENTITY DISORDER (MULTIPLE PERSONALITY DISORDER)

Personality involves the integration of one's thoughts, feelings, and behavior into a sense of unique self. Patients with dissociative identity disorder have two or more distinct personalities that alternately control their behaviors and thoughts. Patients are often unable to recall personal information. While one personality is dominant, that personality is usually (but not always) unaware of events that occurred during prior personality states.

DIAGNOSIS AND DSM-IV CRITERIA

- Presence of two or more distinct identities
- At least two of the identities recurrently take control of the person's behavior.
- Inability to recall personal information of one personality when the other is dominant
- Not due to effects of substance or medical condition

EPIDEMIOLOGY

- Women account for more than 90% of patients.
- Most patients have experienced prior trauma, especially childhood physical or sexual abuse.
- Average age of diagnosis is 30.
- High incidence of comorbid major depression, anxiety disorders, borderline personality disorder, and substance abuse. Up to one third of patients attempt suicide.

COURSE AND PROGNOSIS

- Course is usually chronic with incomplete recovery.
- Worst prognosis of all dissociative disorders
- Patients with an earlier onset have a poorer prognosis.

TREATMENT

Hypnosis, drug-assisted interviewing, and insight-oriented psychotherapy; pharmacotherapy as needed if comorbid disorder develops (such as major depression)

▶ DEPERSONALIZATION DISORDER

Depersonalization disorder is characterized by persistent or recurrent feelings of detachment from one's self, environment (derealization), or social situation. Patients feel separated from their bodies and mental processes, as if they are outside observers. They are aware of their symptoms and often fear they are going crazy. Depersonalization is often accompanied by anxiety or panic.

Diagnosis requires that episodes be persistent or recurrent, as transient symptoms of depersonalization are common in normal people during times of stress.

DIAGNOSIS AND DSM-IV CRITERIA

- Persistent or recurrent experiences of being detached from one's body or mental processes
- Reality testing remains intact during episode.

A 40-year-old sanitation worker currently lives in Baltimore for the past 2 years. He moved from Miami where he owned a small restaurant for 10 years. When he is approached by a woman who claims to be his former neighbor from Miami, he has no memory of living there or owning a restaurant. *Think: Dissociative fugue.*

Symptoms of multiple personality disorder may be similar to those seen in borderline personality disorder.

A 33-year-old nun is astounded when a man claims that he saw her at a local strip club the night before. She denies his accusations and has no memory of the event. *Think: Dissociative identity disorder (multiple personality disorder).*

A 30-year-old male says that he had an "out of this world" experience. He felt as if "he was watching his own life like a movie." He knows this is not normal. *Think: Depersonalization disorder.*

■ Causes social/occupational impairment, and cannot be accounted for by another mental or physical disorder

EPIDEMIOLOGY

■ Approximately twice as common in women than men
■ Average onset between ages 15 and 30
■ Increased incidence of comorbid anxiety disorders and major depression
■ Severe stress is a predisposing factor.

COURSE AND PROGNOSIS

Often chronic (with either steady or intermittent course), but may remit without treatment

TREATMENT

Antianxiety agents or selective serotonin reuptake inhibitors (SSRIs) to treat associated symptoms of anxiety or major depression

Somatoform Disorders and Factitious Disorders

> ## ▶ DEFINITION

Patients with somatoform disorders present with physical symptoms that have no organic cause. They truly believe that their symptoms are due to medical problems and are not consciously feigning symptoms.

Examples of somatoform disorders include:
- Somatization disorder
- Conversion disorder
- Hypochondriasis
- Pain disorder
- Body dysmorphic disorder

Primary and secondary gain often result from symptoms expressed in somatoform disorders, but patients are not consciously aware of gains and do not intentionally seek them.

Primary gain: Expression of unacceptable feelings as physical symptoms in order to avoid facing them

Secondary gain: Use of symptoms to benefit the patient (increased attention from others, decreased responsibilities, avoidance of the law, etc.).

With the exception of hypochondriasis, somatoform disorders are more common in women. One half of patients have comorbid mental disorders, especially anxiety disorders and major depression.

When suspecting a somatoform disorder, one must always rule out organic causes of symptoms, including central nervous system (CNS) disease, endocrine disorders, and connective tissue disorders.

> ## ▶ SOMATIZATION DISORDER

Patients with somatization disorder present with multiple vague complaints involving many organ systems. They have a long-standing history of numerous visits to doctors. Their symptoms cannot be explained by a medical disorder.

DIAGNOSIS AND DSM-IV CRITERIA

- At least two gastrointestinal (GI) symptoms
- At least one sexual or reproductive symptom

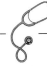

Five to 10% of patients presenting in primary care have a somatization disorder.

Somatization—**So many** physical complaints

- At least one neurological symptom
- At least four pain symptoms
- Onset **before age 30**
- Cannot be explained by general medical condition or substance use

EPIDEMIOLOGY

- Incidence in females 5 to 20 times that of males
- Lifetime prevalence: 0.1 to 0.5%
- Greater prevalence in low socioeconomic groups
- Fifty percent have comorbid mental disorder.
- First-degree female relatives have 10 to 20% incidence.
- 30% concordance in identical twins

COURSE AND PROGNOSIS

Usually chronic and debilitating. Symptoms may periodically improve and then worsen under stress.

TREATMENT

There is no cure, but management involves regularly scheduled frequent visits to a primary care practitioner, since these patients will usually not agree to see a psychiatrist. Secondary gain should be minimized. Medications should be used with caution and only with a clear indication; they are usually ineffective, and patients tend to be erratic in their use. Relaxation therapy, hypnosis, and individual and group psychotherapy are sometimes helpful.

A middle-aged woman presents to her primary care doctor with numerous symptoms involving several organ systems. She has been unwell or "sickly" since early adulthood or adolescence and describes herself as suffering. She is resistant to psychiatric referral. *Think: Somatization disorder.*

▶ **CONVERSION DISORDER**

Patients have at least one neurological symptom (sensory or motor) that cannot be explained by a medical disorder. Onset is always preceded or exacerbated by a psychological stressor, although the patient may not connect the two. Patients are often surprisingly calm and unconcerned (*la belle indifference*) when describing their symptoms, which may include blindness or paralysis.

DIAGNOSIS AND DSM-IV CRITERIA

Conversion disorder: Patients **convert** psychiatric problems to a neurological problem and then spontaneously **convert** back to normal.

- At least one neurological symptom
- Psychological factors associated with initiation or exacerbation of symptom
- Symptom not intentionally produced
- Cannot be explained by medical condition or substance use
- Causes significant distress or impairment in social or occupational functioning
- Not accounted for by somatization disorder or other mental disorder
- Not limited to pain or sexual symptom

Common Symptoms
- Shifting paralysis
- Blindness
- Mutism
- Paresthesias
- Seizures
- Globus hystericus (sensation of lump in throat)

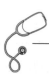

If conversion-like presentation is in older age, it is more likely a neurological deficit.

EPIDEMIOLOGY

- Common disorder
- 20 to 25% incidence in general medical settings
- Two to five times more common in women than men
- Onset at any age, but most often in adolescence or early adulthood
- Increased incidence in low socioeconomic groups
- High incidence of comorbid schizophrenia, major depression, or anxiety disorders

DIFFERENTIAL DIAGNOSIS

Must rule out underlying medical cause, as 50% of these patients eventually receive medical diagnoses

COURSE

Symptoms resolve within 1 month. Twenty-five percent will eventually have future episodes, especially during times of stress. Symptoms may spontaneously resolve after hypnosis or **sodium amobarbital** interview if the psychological trigger can be uncovered during the interview.

TREATMENT

Insight-oriented psychotherapy, hypnosis, or relaxation therapy if needed. Most patients spontaneously recover.

▶ HYPOCHONDRIASIS

Hypochondriasis involves prolonged, exaggerated concern about health and possible illness. Patients either fear having a disease or are convinced that one is present. They misinterpret normal bodily symptoms as indicative of disease.

DIAGNOSIS AND DSM-IV CRITERIA

- Patients fear that they have a serious medical condition based on misinterpretation of normal body symptoms.
- Fears persist despite appropriate medical evaluation.
- Fears present for at least **6 months**

EPIDEMIOLOGY

- Men affected as often as women
- Average age of onset: 20 to 30
- Eighty percent have coexisting major depression or anxiety disorder.

DIFFERENTIAL DIAGNOSIS

- Must rule out underlying medical condition
- *Somatization disorder*—hypochondriacs are worried about *disease*, whereas patients with somatization disorder are concerned about their *symptoms*.

COURSE

Episodic—symptoms may wax and wane periodically. Exacerbations occur commonly under stress. Up to 50% of patients improve significantly.

A 20-year-old woman visits her doctor stating that she has been blind since the previous day. She seems calm and indifferent. The blindness began 1 week following her son's death. Her neurological exam is normal, and nerve studies reveal no retinal problems. *Think: Conversion disorder.*

A 30-year-old male visits the medical clinic with concerns about colon cancer. He has had intermittent abdominal pain for the past year and has seen several doctors. He had a normal upper GI series, colonoscopy, and computed tomography (CT) scan. After each test came back normal, he was initially reassured but then began worrying again a short time later. On this visit, copies of his prior evaluations and physical exams are unremarkable. When he is confronted with the idea of seeing a mental health professional, he storms out of the office and seeks another physician. *Think: Hypochondriasis.*

TREATMENT

No cure exists, but management involves frequently scheduled visits to *one* primary care doctor who oversees the patient's care. Patients are usually resistant to psychotherapy. Group therapy or insight-oriented psychotherapy may be helpful if patient is willing.

A 20-year-old single female visits a plastic surgeon requesting a nose job because her nose is "huge and ugly." She says everyone stares at her because of her repulsive face, so she rarely goes out. On inspection, her nose appears perfectly normal and small. After the procedure, she is unhappy with the result and still insists her nose is large. *Think: Body dysmorphic disorder.*

▶ BODY DYSMORPHIC DISORDER

Patients with body dysmorphic disorder are preoccupied with body parts that they perceive as flawed or defective. Though their physical imperfections are either minimal or completely imagined, patients view them as severe and grotesque. They are extremely self-conscious about their appearance and spend significant time trying to correct perceived flaws with makeup, dermatological procedures, or plastic surgery.

DIAGNOSIS AND DSM-IV CRITERIA

- Preoccupation with an imagined defect in appearance or excessive concern about a slight physical anomaly
- Must cause significant distress in the patient's life

EPIDEMIOLOGY

- More common in women than men
- More common in unmarried than married persons
- Average age of onset: Between 15 and 20
- Ninety percent have coexisting major depression.
- Seventy percent have coexisting anxiety disorder.
- Thirty percent have coexisting psychotic disorder.

COURSE AND PROGNOSIS

Usually chronic; symptoms wax and wane in intensity.

TREATMENT

Surgical or dermatological procedures are routinely unsuccessful in pleasing the patient. Selective serotonin reuptake inhibitors (SSRIs) reduce symptoms in 50% of patients.

▶ PAIN DISORDER

Patients with pain disorder have prolonged, severe discomfort without adequate medical explanation. The pain often co-exists with a medical condition but is not directly caused by it. Patients often have a history of multiple visits to doctors. Pain disorder can be acute (< 6 months) or chronic (> 6 months).

DIAGNOSIS AND DSM-IV CRITERIA

- Patient's main complaint is of pain at one or more anatomic sites.
- The pain causes significant distress in the patient's life.
- The pain has to be related to psychological factors.
- The pain is not due to a true medical disorder.

Epidemiology

- Women are two times as likely as men to have pain disorder.
- Average age of onset: 30 to 50
- Increased incidence in first-degree relatives
- Increased incidence in blue-collar workers
- Patients have higher incidence of major depression, anxiety disorders, and substance abuse.

Differential Diagnosis

- Must rule out underlying medical condition
- Hypochondriasis and malingering

Course

Abrupt onset and increase in intensity for first several months; usually a chronic and disabling course

Treatment

Analgesics are not helpful, and patients often become dependent on them. SSRIs, transient nerve stimulation, biofeedback, hypnosis, and psychotherapy may be beneficial.

A 40-year-old female is referred to an orthopedist for severe ankle pain since a minor ankle injury while playing tennis 10 months ago. Physical exam, x-ray, and magnetic resonance imaging (MRI) reveal no abnormality. *Think: Pain disorder.*

▶ FACTITIOUS DISORDER

Patients with factitious disorder intentionally produce medical or psychological symptoms in order to assume the role of a sick patient. *Primary gain* is a prominent feature of this disorder (see definition p. 105).

Diagnosis and DSM-IV Criteria

- Patients **intentionally** produce signs of physical or mental disorders.
- They produce the symptoms to assume the role of the patient (*primary gain*).
- There are no external incentives (such as monetary reward, etc.)
- Either predominantly psychiatric complaints or predominantly physical complaints

Commonly Feigned Symptoms
- *Psychiatric*—hallucinations, depression
- *Medical*—fever (by heating the thermometer), abdominal pain, seizures, skin lesions, and hematuria

Related Disorders

Münchhausen syndrome—another name for factitious disorder with predominantly physical complaints. These patients may take insulin, consume blood thinners, or mix feces in their urine in order to produce symptoms of medical disease. In addition, they will often demand specific medications. They are very skilled at feigning symptoms necessitating hospitalization.

Münchhausen syndrome by proxy—intentionally producing symptoms in someone else who is under one's care (usually one's children) in order to assume the sick role by proxy

A 30-year-old male medical laboratory assistant is admitted to the hospital for fever and bacteremia. The patient requires a central venous line because of poor venous access. Multiple blood cultures reveal unusual organisms in the blood, and a total of eight different organisms are isolated over the course of his stay. The patient locks himself in the bathroom for extended periods of time, and his room is full of half-empty soda cans. Upon careful inspection of his room, one can is noted to have a syringe in it. When the patient is confronted with the hypothesis that he has been injecting himself with contaminated syringes, he signs out of the hospital. *Think: Factitious disorder.*

EPIDEMIOLOGY

- > 5% of all hospitalized patients
- Increased incidence in males
- Higher incidence in hospital and health care workers (who have learned how to feign symptoms)
- Associated with higher intelligence, poor sense of identity, and poor sexual adjustment

Many patients have a history of child abuse or neglect. Inpatient hospitalization resulting from abuse provided a safe, comforting environment, thus linking the sick role with a positive experience.

COURSE AND PROGNOSIS

Repeated and long-term hospitalizations are common.

TREATMENT

No effective treatment exists, but it is important to avoid unnecessary procedures and to maintain a close liaison with the patient's primary medical doctor. Patients who are confronted while in the hospital usually leave.

A 50-year-old male claims to have headaches, severe back pain, knee pain, and blurry vision since a minor car accident 8 weeks ago. Physical exam and medical workup reveal no abnormalities. After the patient receives a $75,000 settlement, his symptoms disappear.
Think: Malingering.

▶ MALINGERING

Malingering involves the feigning of physical or psychological symptoms in order to achieve personal gain. Common external motivations include avoiding the police, receiving room and board, obtaining narcotics, and receiving monetary compensation.

PRESENTATION

Patients usually present with multiple vague complaints that do not conform to a known medical condition. They often have a long medical history with many hospital stays. They are generally uncooperative and refuse to accept a good prognosis even after extensive medical evaluation. However, their symptoms improve once their desired objective is obtained.

EPIDEMIOLOGY

- Common in hospitalized patients
- More common in men than women

▶ REVIEW OF DISTINGUISHING FEATURES

Somatoform disorders: Patients *believe* they are ill.
Factitious disorders: Patients *pretend* they are ill with no obvious external reward.
Malingering (most common): Patients pretend they are ill with obvious *external incentive.*

Impulse Control Disorders

Impulse control disorders are characterized by an *inability to resist* behaviors that may bring harm to oneself or to others. Patients may or may not try to suppress their impulses and may not feel remorse or guilt after they have acted out. *Anxiety* or tension is often experienced prior to the impulse, and *relief* or satisfaction results after the behavior is completed.

Impulse control disorders are not caused by another mental condition, general medical problem, or substance use.

▶ **INTERMITTENT EXPLOSIVE DISORDER**

DIAGNOSIS AND DSM-IV CRITERIA

- Failure to resist aggressive impulses that result in assault or property destruction
- Level of aggressiveness is out of proportion to any triggering events

Individual episodes of explosive behavior often remit quickly and spontaneously, and patients usually feel remorseful.

EPIDEMIOLOGY/ETIOLOGY

- More common in men than women
- Onset usually late teens or twenties
- Genetic, perinatal, environmental, and neurobiological factors may play a role in etiology. Patients may have history of child abuse, head trauma, or seizures.
- May progress in severity until middle age

TREATMENT

Treatment involves use of selective serotonin reuptake inhibitors (SSRIs), anticonvulsants, lithium, and propanolol. Individual psychotherapy is difficult and ineffective. Group therapy and/or family therapy may be useful.

Low levels of serotonin have been shown to be associated with impulsiveness and aggression.

▶ KLEPTOMANIA

DIAGNOSIS AND DSM-IV CRITERIA

- Failure to resist urges to steal objects that are not needed for personal or monetary reasons
- Pleasure or relief is experienced while stealing
- Purpose of stealing is not to express anger and is not due to a hallucination or delusion

EPIDEMIOLOGY/ETIOLOGY

- More common in women than men
- Occurs in under 5% of shoplifters
- Symptoms often occur during times of stress.
- Increased incidence of comorbid mood disorders, eating disorders, and obsessive–compulsive disorder
- Etiology may involve biological factors and childhood family dysfunction
- Course is usually chronic.

One fourth of patients with bulimia nervosa have comorbid kleptomania.

TREATMENT

Treatment may include insight-oriented psychotherapy, behavior therapy (systematic desensitization and aversive conditioning), and SSRIs. There is some anecdotal evidence for naltrexone use.

▶ PYROMANIA

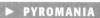

DIAGNOSIS AND DSM-IV CRITERIA

- More than one episode of intentional fire setting
- Tension present before the act and pleasure or relief experienced afterwards
- Fascination with or attraction to fire and its uses and consequences
- Purpose of fire setting not for monetary gain, expression of anger, making a political statement, and is not due to a hallucination or delusion

EPIDEMIOLOGY/ETIOLOGY

- More common in men and mentally retarded individuals
- Prognosis better in children than adults (with treatment, children often recover completely)

TREATMENT

Treatment involves use of behavior therapy, supervision, and SSRIs.

DIAGNOSIS AND DSM-IV CRITERIA

Recurrent maladaptive gambling behavior, as shown by five or more of the following:

1. Preoccupation with gambling
2. Need to gamble with increasing amount of money to achieve pleasure
3. Repeated and unsuccessful attempts to cut down on gambling
4. Restlessness or irritability when attempting to stop gambling
5. Gambling done to escape problems or relieve dysphoria
6. Returning to reclaim losses after gambling
7. Lying to therapist or family members to hide level of gambling
8. Committing illegal acts to finance gambling
9. Jeopardizing relationships or job because of gambling
10. Relying on others to financially support gambling

EPIDEMIOLOGY/ETIOLOGY

- Prevalence: 1 to 3% of U.S. adults
- More common in men than women
- Increased incidence of mood disorders, anxiety disorders, and obsessive–compulsive disorder
- Predisposing factors include loss of a parent during childhood, inappropriate parental discipline during childhood, attention deficit hyperactivity disorder, and lack of family emphasis on budgeting or saving money.
- Etiology may involve genetic, biological, environmental, and neurochemical factors.

TREATMENT

Participation in Gamblers Anonymous (a 12-step program) is the most effective treatment. After 3 months of abstinence from gambling, insight-oriented psychotherapy may be attempted. It is also important to treat comorbid mood disorders, anxiety disorders, and substance abuse problems.

DIAGNOSIS AND DSM-IV CRITERIA

- Recurrent pulling out of one's hair, resulting in visible hair loss
- Usually involves scalp, but can involve eyebrows, eyelashes, and facial and pubic hair
- Tension present before the behavior, and pleasure or relief resulting afterwards
- Causes significant distress or impairment in daily functioning

EPIDEMIOLOGY/ETIOLOGY

- Seen in 1 to 3% of the population
- More common in women than men
- Onset usually during childhood or adolescence and occurs after stressful event in one fourth of patients

- Etiology may involve biological factors, genetic factors, and environmental factors (such as problems in relationship with mother, recent loss of important object or figure, etc.)
- Increased incidence of co-morbid obsessive–compulsive disorder, obsessive–compulsive personality disorder, mood disorders, and borderline personality disorder
- Course may be chronic or remitting; adult onset generally more difficult to treat

TREATMENT

- SSRIs, antipsychotics, lithium
- Hypnosis, relaxation techniques
- Behavioral therapy, including substituting another behavior and/or positive reinforcement (viewing hair pulling as simply a habit)

Eating Disorders

► DEFINITION

Eating disorders include anorexia nervosa, bulimia nervosa, and binge-eating disorder. Patients with anorexia or bulimia have a disturbed body image and use extensive measures to avoid gaining weight (vomiting, laxatives, excessive exercise, etc.). Binge eating may occur in all of the eating disorders.

► ANOREXIA NERVOSA

Patients with anorexia nervosa are preoccupied with their weight, their body image, and with being thin. There are two main subdivisions:
- *Restrictive type:* Eat very little and may vigorously exercise; more often withdrawn with obsessive–compulsive traits
- *Binge eating/purging type:* Eat in binges followed by purging, laxatives, excessive exercise, and/or diuretics; associated with increased incidence of major depression and substance abuse

DIAGNOSIS AND DSM-IV CRITERIA

- Body weight at least 15% below normal
- Intense fear of gaining weight or becoming fat
- Disturbed body image
- Amenorrhea

PHYSICAL FINDINGS AND COMPLICATIONS

Amenorrhea, electrolyte abnormalities (hypochloremic hyperkalemic alkalosis), hypercholesterolemia, arrhythmias, cardiac arrest, lanugo (fine body hair), melanosis coli (darkened area of colon secondary to laxative abuse), leukopenia, osteoporosis

EPIDEMIOLOGY

- 10 to 20 times more common in women than men
- Occurs in up to 4% of adolescents and young adults (mainly females)
- Onset usually between ages 10 and 30

Anorexia nervosa involves **low body weight,** and this distinguishes it from bulimia.

Extremely thin, amenorrheic teenage girl whose mother says she eats very little, does aerobics for 2 hours a day, and *ritualistically* does 400 sit-ups every day (500 if she has "overeaten")
Think: Anorexia nervosa.

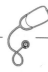

Anorexia Versus Major Depression

Anorexia nervosa: Patients have *good appetite* but starve themselves due to distorted body image. They are often quite preoccupied with food, preparing it for others, etc., but do not eat it themselves.

Major depression: Patients usually have *poor appetite*, which leads to weight loss. These patients have no interest in food.

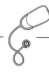

Unlike patients with anorexia nervosa, bulimic patients usually maintain a **normal weight,** and their symptoms are more **ego-dystonic** (distressing); they are therefore more likely to seek help.

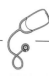

Binge eating is defined by excessive food intake within a 2-hour period accompanied by a sense of lack of control.

- More common in developed countries and professions requiring thin physique (such as ballet or modeling)
- Etiology involves environmental, social, biological, and genetic factors
- Increased incidence of comorbid mood disorders

DIFFERENTIAL DIAGNOSIS

Medical condition (such as cancer), major depression, bulimia, or other mental disorder (such as somatization disorder or schizophrenia)

COURSE AND PROGNOSIS

- Variable course—may completely recover, have fluctuating symptoms with relapses, or progressively deteriorate
- Mortality approximately 10% due to starvation, suicide, or electrolyte disturbance

TREATMENT

Patients may be treated as outpatients unless they are more than 20% below ideal body weight, in which case they should be hospitalized.

Treatment involves behavioral therapy, family therapy, and supervised weight-gain programs. Some antidepressants may be useful as adjunctive treatment to promote weight gain, such as paroxetine or mirtazapine. Others promote weight *loss*, so it is important to check side effect profiles before prescribing.

▶ BULIMIA NERVOSA

Bulimia nervosa involves binge eating combined with behaviors intended to counteract weight gain, such as vomiting, use of laxatives or diuretics, or excessive exercise. Patients are embarrassed by their bingeing and are overly concerned with body weight. However, unlike patients with anorexia, they usually maintain a normal weight (and may be overweight).

There are two subcategories of bulimia:
- *Purging type*—involves vomiting, laxatives, or diuretics
- *Nonpurging type*—involves excessive exercise or fasting

DIAGNOSIS AND DSM-IV CRITERIA

- Recurrent episodes of binge eating
- Recurrent, inappropriate attempts to compensate for overeating and prevent weight gain (such as laxative abuse, vomiting, diuretics, or excessive exercise)
- The binge eating and compensatory behaviors occur at least twice a week for 3 months.
- Perception of self-worth is excessively influenced by body weight and shape.

PHYSICAL FINDINGS AND COMPLICATIONS

Hypochloremic hypokalemic alkalosis (with or without arrhythmias), esophagitis, dental erosion, calloused knuckles (from self-induced vomiting), and salivary gland hypertrophy

EPIDEMIOLOGY

- Affects 1 to 3% of adolescent and young females
- Significantly more common in women than men
- More common in developed countries
- High incidence of comorbid mood disorders, impulse control disorders, and alcohol abuse/dependence

COURSE AND PROGNOSIS

- Better prognosis than anorexia nervosa
- Symptoms usually exacerbated by stressful conditions
- One half recover fully with treatment; one half have chronic course with fluctuating symptoms

TREATMENT

Treatment may include individual psychotherapy, cognitive–behavioral therapy, group therapy, and pharmacotherapy (selective serotonin reuptake inhibitors [SSRIs] are first-line, then tricyclic antidepressants [TCAs]).

A 20-year-old college student is referred by her dentist because of multiple dental caries. She is normal for her weight but feels that "she needs to lose 15 pounds." She reluctantly admits to eating a large quantity of food in a short period of time and then inducing gagging. *Think: Bulimia nervosa.*

▶ BINGE-EATING DISORDER

Obesity is defined as being at least 20% over ideal body weight. Over one half of all people in the United States are obese. Genetic factors, overeating, and lack of activity may all contribute to the development of obesity. Excess weight is associated with adverse effects on health, including increased risk of diabetes, hypertension, cardiac disease, and osteoarthritis.

Binge-eating disorder falls under the DSM-IV category of Eating Disorder NOS (not otherwise specified). Patients with this disorder suffer emotional distress over their binge eating, but they do not try to control their weight by purging or restricting calories, as do anorexics or bulimics.

DIAGNOSIS AND DSM-IV CRITERIA

- Recurrent episodes of binge eating (eating an excessive amount of food in a 2-hour period associated with a lack of control)
- Severe distress over binge eating
- Bingeing occurs at least 2 days a week for 6 months and is not associated with compensatory behaviors (such as vomiting, laxative use, etc.)
- Three or more of the following are present:
  1. Eating very rapidly
  2. Eating until uncomfortably full
  3. Eating large amounts when not hungry
  4. Eating alone due to embarrassment over eating habits
  5. Feeling disgusted, depressed, or guilty after overeating

TREATMENT

Treatment involves individual psychotherapy and behavioral therapy with a strict diet and exercise program. Comorbid mood disorders or anxiety disorders should be treated as necessary.

Pharmacotherapy may be used adjunctively to promote weight loss, including:

- Stimulants (such as phentermine and amphetamine)—suppress appetite
- Orlistat (Xenical)—inhibits pancreatic lipase, thus decreasing amount of fat absorbed from gastrointestinal tract
- Sibutramine (Meridia)—inhibits reuptake of norepinephrine, serotonin, and dopamine

Sleep Disorders

Sleep disorders are very common in the general population. Up to one third of people in the United States will experience a sleep disorder at some point in their lives. Causes of sleep disorders include:

- Medical conditions (pain, metabolic disorders, endocrine disorders, etc.)
- Physical conditions (obesity, etc.)
- Sedative withdrawal
- Use of stimulants (caffeine, amphetamines, etc.)
- Major depression (causes early morning awakening or hypersomnia)
- Mania or anxiety
- Neurotransmitter abnormalities:
    - Elevated dopamine or norepinephrine causes decreased total sleep time
    - Elevated acetylcholine causes increased total sleep time and increased proportion of rapid eye movement (REM) sleep
    - Elevated serotonin causes increased total sleep time and increased proportion of delta wave sleep

Sleep disorders are classified as either *primary* (not due to another medical condition or substance use) or *secondary* (due to another medical condition or substance use).

Primary sleep disorders may be further subdivided into:

1. **Dyssomnias**—disturbances in the amount, quality, or timing of sleep
2. **Parasomnias**—abnormal events in behavior or physiology during sleep

See Table 15-1.

TABLE 15-1. Normal Sleep Cycle

Stage	EEG Wave Type	% of Sleep
I. Non-REM Sleep		75%
Eyes *open*, awake	Mixed frequency, desynchronized	
Eyes *closed*, awake	Alpha waves (12% of people do not have alpha waves)	
Stage 1—Lightest sleep	Loss of alpha waves	5%
Stage 2—Light sleep	Sleep spindles and k-complexes	45%
Stage 3–4—Deep sleep (most restorative)	Delta waves (lowest frequency)	25%
II. REM Sleep		25%
Cycles last 10–40 minutes and occur every 90 minutes; involve dreaming, lack of motor tone, erections.	Sawtooth waves Rapid eye movement	
Amount of REM sleep decreases with age.		
REM rebound is an increase in amount of REM sleep that occurs after a night of sleep deprivation. Slow-wave sleep is made up first.		

When evaluating insomnia, be sure to ask about daily caffeine intake—both quantity and the times of day it is ingested.

A 40-year-old businessman states that over the past 2 years, he has trouble staying awake for more than 2 hours before falling asleep. He has a hard time sleeping through the night. Meanwhile, his performance at work is suffering. *Think: Primary insomnia.*

▶ DYSSOMNIAS

Primary Insomnia

DIAGNOSIS

Difficulty initiating or maintaining sleep, resulting in daytime drowsiness or difficulty fulfilling tasks. Disturbance occurs three or more times per week for at least 1 month.

EPIDEMIOLOGY/ETIOLOGY

- Affects 30% of the general population
- Often exacerbated by anxiety and preoccupation with getting enough sleep

TREATMENT

1. Sleep hygiene measures (first line):
   - Maintain regular sleep schedule.
   - Limit caffeine intake.
   - Avoid daytime naps.
   - Exercise early in day.
   - Soak in hot tub prior to bedtime.
   - Avoid large meals near bedtime.
   - Remove disturbances such as TV and telephone from bedroom (bedroom for sleep and sex only).
2. Pharmacotherapy (for short-term use): Benadryl, Ambien (zolpidem), Sonata (zaleplon), Desyrel (trazodone)

Primary Hypersomnia

DIAGNOSIS

- At least 1 month of excessive daytime sleepiness or excessive sleep not attributable to medical condition, medications, poor sleep hygiene, insufficient sleep, or narcolepsy
- Usually begins in adolescence

TREATMENT

- Stimulant drugs (amphetamines) are first line.
- Selective serotonin reuptake inhibitors (SSRIs) may be useful in some patients.

Narcolepsy

DIAGNOSIS

Repeated, sudden attacks of sleep in the daytime for at least 3 months, associated with:

1. *Cataplexy*—collapse due to sudden loss of muscle tone (occurs in 70% of patients); associated with emotion, particularly laughter
2. Short REM latency
3. Sleep paralysis—brief paralysis upon awakening (in 50% of patients)
4. Hypnagogic (as patient falls asleep or is falling asleep); hypnopompic (as patient wakes up; dream persists); hallucinations (in approximately 30% of patients)

EPIDEMIOLOGY/ETIOLOGY

- Occurs in 0.02 to 0.16% of adult population
- Equal incidence in males and females
- Onset most commonly during childhood or adolescence
- May have genetic component
- Patients usually have poor nighttime sleep

TREATMENT

Timed daily naps plus stimulant drugs (amphetamines and methylphenidate). SSRIs or sodium oxalate for cataplexy.

Breathing-Related Disorders

DIAGNOSIS

Sleep disruption and excessive daytime sleepiness (EDS) caused by abnormal sleep ventilation from either obstructive or central sleep apnea

EPIDEMIOLOGY

- Up to 10% of adults
- More common in men and obese persons
- Associated with headaches, depression, pulmonary hypertension, and sudden death in elderly and infants
- Obstructive sleep apnea (OSA): Strong correlation with snoring
- Central sleep apnea (CSA) correlated with heart failure

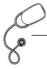

Although benzodiazepines are effective hypnotics, avoid use if possible due to risk of dependence.

A 30-year-old woman says that despite getting an adequate amount of sleep during the night, she has trouble staying awake at work. During her lunch hour, she goes to the lounge and takes a nap, which does not refresh her. In the morning, she has trouble getting out of bed and is often confused. *Think: Primary hypersomnia.*

A 20-year-old college student complains that over the past 4 months, he falls asleep "out of the blue" in the daytime and then has trouble moving his body on awakening. He gets 9 hours of restless sleep every night and denies any substance abuse or significant medical illnesses. *Think: Narcolepsy.*

Two Concepts to Distinguish EDS vs. Fatigue: EDS is falling asleep when you don't want to (e.g., near misses while driving, at a stop light, after a large meal). This is common with OSA.
Fatigue is being too tired to complete activities.

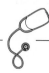

Obstructive sleep apnea—respiratory effort is present, but ventilation disrupted by physical obstruction of airflow

Versus

Central sleep apnea—periodic cessation of respiratory effort

A 50-year-old obese male with hypertension states that he feels very tired and sleepy throughout the day despite getting an adequate amount of sleep during the nighttime. His wife tells you that even she has trouble sleeping due to his loud snoring. *Think: Obstructive sleep apnea.*

OSA Risk Factors

- Male gender
- Obesity
- Male shirt collar size ≥ 17
- Prior upper airway surgeries
- Deviated nasal septum
- "Kissing" tonsils
- Large uvula, tongue
- Retrognathia

Treatment

OSA: Nasal continuous positive airway pressure (nCPAP), weight loss, nasal surgery, or uvulopalatoplasty
CSA: Mechanical ventilation (such as b-PAP) with a backup rate

Circadian Rhythm Sleep Disorder

Diagnosis

Disturbance of sleep due to mismatch between circadian sleep–wake cycle and environmental sleep demands. Subtypes include jet lag type, shift work type, and delayed sleep or advanced sleep phase type.

Treatment

- Jet lag type usually remits untreated after 2 to 7 days
- Light therapy may be useful for shift work type
- For shift life, delayed/advanced phase is better
- Melatonin can be given 5½ hrs before desired bedtime

▶ **PARASOMNIAS**

Nightmare Disorder

Diagnosis

- Repeated awakenings with recall of extremely frightening dreams
- Occurs during REM sleep and causes significant distress

Epidemiology

- Onset most often in childhood
- May occur more frequently during times of stress or illness

Treatment

Usually none, but tricyclics or other agents that suppress total REM sleep may be used

Night Terror Disorder

DIAGNOSIS

Repeated episodes of apparent fearfulness during sleep, usually beginning with a scream and associated with intense anxiety. Episodes usually occur during the first third of the night during stage 3 or 4 sleep (non-REM). Patients are not awake and do not remember the episodes.

EPIDEMIOLOGY/ETIOLOGY

- Usually occurs in children
- More common in boys than girls
- Prevalence: 1 to 6% of children
- Tends to run in families
- High association with comorbid sleepwalking disorder

TREATMENT

Usually none, but small doses of diazepam at bedtime may be effective (if necessary)

Sleepwalking Disorder (Somnambulism)

DIAGNOSIS

Repeated episodes of getting out of bed and walking, associated with blank stare and difficulty being awakened. Other motor activity may occur, such as getting dressed, talking, or screaming. Behavior usually terminates with patient returning to bed, but patient may awaken with confusion for several minutes. Episodes occur during the first third of the night during stages 3 and 4 sleep and are never remembered.

EPIDEMIOLOGY/ETIOLOGY

- Onset usually between ages 4 and 8; peak prevalence at age 12
- More common in boys than girls and tends to run in families

TREATMENT

Measures to prevent injury in surrounding environment

Unlike patients with night terror disorder or sleepwalking disorder, patients with nightmare disorder fully awaken and remember the episode.

Sexual Disorders

▶ SEXUAL RESPONSE CYCLE

There are several stages of normal sexual response in men and women:

1. *Desire:* The interest in sexual activity
2. *Excitement:* Begins with either fantasy or physical contact. It is characterized in men by erections and in women by vaginal lubrication, clitoral erection, labial swelling, and elevation of the uterus in the pelvis (*tenting*). Both men and women experience nipple erection and increased pulse and blood pressure.
3. *Plateau:* Characterized in men by increased size of the testicles, tightening of the scrotal sac, and secretion of a few drops of seminal fluid. Women experience contraction of the outer one third of the vagina and enlargement of the upper one third of the vagina. Facial flushing and increases in pulse, blood pressure, and respiration occur in both men and women.
4. *Orgasm:* Men ejaculate and women have contractions of the uterus and lower one third of the vagina.
5. *Resolution:* Muscles relax and cardiovascular state returns to baseline. Men have a *refractory period* during which they cannot be brought to orgasm; women have little or no refractory period.

▶ SEXUAL CHANGES WITH AGING

The desire for sexual activity does not usually change as people age. However, men usually require more direct stimulation of genitals and more time to achieve orgasm. The intensity of ejaculation usually decreases, and the length of refractory period increases.

After menopause, women experience vaginal dryness and thinning due to decreased levels of estrogen. These conditions can be treated with hormone replacement therapy or vaginal creams.

Problems with sexual functioning may be due to any of the following:

1. General medical conditions: Examples include history of atherosclerosis (causing erectile dysfunction from vascular occlusion), diabetes (causing erectile dysfunction from vascular changes and peripheral neuropathy), and pelvic adhesions (causing dyspareunia in women).
2. Abnormal levels of gonadal hormones:
   - *Estrogen*—decreased levels after menopause cause vaginal dryness and thinning in women (without affecting desire).
   - *Testosterone*—promotes libido (desire) in both men and women.
   - *Progesterone*—inhibits libido in both men and women by blocking androgen receptors; found in oral contraceptives, hormone replacement therapy, and treatments for prostate cancer.
3. Medication side effects: antihypertensives, anticholinergics, antidepressants (especially selective serotonin reuptake inhibitors [SSRIs]), and antipsychotics (block dopamine) may contribute to sexual dysfunction.
4. Substance abuse: Alcohol and marijuana enhance sexual desire by suppressing inhibitions. (However, *long-term* alcohol use *decreases* sexual desire.) Cocaine and amphetamines enhance libido by stimulating dopamine receptors. Narcotics inhibit libido.
5. Presence of a sexual disorder (see below).
6. Depression.

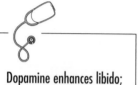

Dopamine enhances libido; serotonin inhibits libido.

Sexual disorders are problems involving any stage of the sexual response cycle. They all share the following DSM-IV criteria:
- The disorder causes marked distress or interpersonal difficulty.
- The dysfunction is not caused by substance use or a general medical condition.

The most common sexual disorders in women are sexual desire disorder and orgasmic disorder. The most common disorders in men are secondary erectile disorder and premature ejaculation. Psychological causes of sexual disorders include:
- Interpersonal problems with sexual partner
- Guilt about sexual activity (often in persons with religious or puritanical upbringing)
- Fears (pregnancy, rejection, loss of control, etc.)

Problems with sexual desire may be due to stress, hostility toward a partner, poor self-esteem, abstinence from sex for a prolonged period, or unconscious fears about sex.

Disorders of Desire

- *Hypoactive sexual desire disorder*—absence or deficiency of sexual desire or fantasies (occurs in up to 20% of general population and is more common in women)
- *Sexual aversion disorder*—avoidance of genital contact with a sexual partner

HIGH-YIELD FACTS

Sexual Disorders

Disorders of Arousal (Excitement and Plateau)

Stress, fear, fatigue, anxiety, and feelings of guilt may contribute to both erectile disorder in men and sexual arousal disorder in women.

- *Male erectile disorder*—inability to attain an erection. May be *primary* (never had one) or *secondary* (acquired after previous ability to maintain erections). Secondary erectile disorder is common and occurs in 10 to 20% of men.
- *Female sexual arousal disorder*—inability to maintain lubrication until completion of sex act (high prevalence—up to 33% of women)

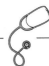

Male erectile disorder is commonly referred to as *impotence.* In men who have erections in the morning and during masturbation, the etiology is usually psychological rather than physical.

Disorders of Orgasm

Both male and female orgasmic disorders may be either *primary* (never achieved orgasm) or *secondary* (acquired). Causes may include relationship problems, guilt, stress, and so on.

- *Female orgasmic disorder:* Inability to have an orgasm after a normal excitement phase. The estimated prevalence in women is 30%.
- *Male orgasmic disorder:* Achieves orgasm with great difficulty, if at all; much lower incidence than impotence or premature ejaculation
- *Premature ejaculation:* Ejaculation earlier than desired time (before or immediately upon entering the vagina). High prevalence—up to 35% of all male sexual disorders; may be caused by fears, guilt, or performance anxiety

In young, sexually inexperienced men (who have shorter refractory periods), premature ejaculation disorder may resolve gradually over time without treatment.

Sexual Pain Disorders

- *Dyspareunia:* Genital pain before, during, or after sexual intercourse; much higher incidence in women than men; often associated with vaginismus (see below)
- *Vaginismus:* Involuntary muscle contraction of the outer third of the vagina during insertion of penis or object (such as speculum or tampon); increased incidence in higher socioeconomic groups and in women of strict religious upbringing

▶ TREATMENT OF SEXUAL DISORDERS

Dual Sex Therapy

Dual sex therapy utilizes the concept of the marital unit, rather than the individual, as the target of therapy. Couples meet with a male and female therapist together in four-way sessions to identify and discuss their sexual problems. Therapists suggest sexual exercises for the couple to attempt at home; activities initially focus on heightening sensory awareness and progressively incorporate increased levels of sexual contact. Treatment is short term.

Behavior Therapy

Behavior therapy approaches sexual dysfunction as a learned maladaptive behavior. It utilizes traditional therapies such as systematic desensitization, where patients are progressively exposed to increasing levels of stimuli that provoke their anxiety. Eventually, patients are able to respond appropriately to the stimuli. Other forms of behavioral therapy include muscle relaxation techniques, assertiveness training, and prescribed sexual exercises to try at home.

Hypnosis

Most often used adjunctively with other therapies

Group Therapy

May be used as primary or adjunctive therapy

Analytically Oriented Psychotherapy

Individual, long-term therapy that focuses on feelings, fears, dreams, and interpersonal problems that may be contributing to sexual disorder

Others

Specific techniques for various dysfunctions:

Sexual desire disorder: Testosterone (if levels are low)

Erectile disorder: Yohimbine, sildenafil (Viagra), self-injection of vasoactive substances (such as alprostadil), vacuum pumps, constrictive rings, prosthetic surgery (last resort)

Female sexual arousal disorder: Release of clitoral adhesions (if necessary)

Male orgasmic disorder: Gradual progression from extravaginal ejaculation (via masturbation) to intravaginal

Female orgasmic disorder: Masturbation (sometimes with vibrator)

Premature ejaculation:

- The *squeeze technique* is used to increase the threshold of excitability. When the man has been excited to near ejaculation, he or his sexual partner is instructed to squeeze the glans of his penis in order to prevent ejaculation. Gradually, he gains awareness about his sexual sensations and learns to achieve greater ejaculatory control.
- The *stop–start technique* involves cessation of all penile stimulation when the man is near ejaculation. This technique functions in the same manner as the squeeze technique.
- Pharmacotherapy: Side effects of drugs including SSRIs and tricyclics may prolong sexual response.

Dyspareunia: Gradual desensitization to achieve intercourse, starting with muscle relaxation techniques, progressing to erotic massage, and finally achieving sexual intercourse

Vaginismus: Women may obtain some relief by dilating their vaginas regularly with their fingers or a dilator.

Paraphilias are sexual disorders characterized by engagement in unusual sexual activities (and/or preoccupation with unusual sexual urges or fantasies) for at least 6 months that cause impairment in daily functioning. Paraphilic fantasies alone are not considered disorders unless they are intense, recurrent, and interfere with daily life; occasional fantasies are considered normal components of sexuality (even if unusual).

Only a small percentage of people suffer from paraphilias. Most paraphilias occur only in men, but sadism, masochism, and pedophilia may also occur in women. The most common paraphilias are pedophilia, voyeurism, and exhibitionism.

Examples of Paraphilias

- **Pedophilia:** Sexual gratification from fantasies or behaviors involving sexual acts with children (most common paraphilia)
- **Voyeurism:** Watching unsuspecting nude individuals (often with binoculars) in order to obtain sexual pleasure
- **Exhibitionism:** Exposure of one's genitals to strangers
- **Fetishism:** Sexual preference for inanimate objects (e.g., shoes or pantyhose)
- **Transvestic fetishism:** Sexual gratification in men (usually heterosexual) from wearing women's clothing (especially underwear)
- **Frotteurism:** Sexual pleasure in men from rubbing their genitals against unsuspecting women; usually occurs in a crowded area (such as subway)
- **Masochism:** Sexual excitement from being humiliated or beaten
- **Sadism:** Sexual excitement from hurting or humiliating another
- **Necrophilia:** Sexual pleasure from engaging in sexual activity with dead people
- **Telephone scatologia:** Sexual excitement from calling unsuspecting women and engaging in sexual conversations with them

COURSE AND PROGNOSIS

Poor prognostic factors are early age of onset, comorbid substance abuse, high frequency of behavior, and referral by law enforcement agencies (after arrest).

Good prognostic factors are self-referral for treatment, sense of guilt associated with the behavior, and history of otherwise normal sexual activity in addition to the paraphilia.

TREATMENT

- **Insight-oriented psychotherapy:** Most common method. Patients gain insight into the stimuli that cause them to act as they do.
- **Behavior therapy:** Aversive conditioning used to disrupt the learned abnormal behavior by coupling the impulse with an unpleasant stimulus such as an electric shock.
- **Pharmacologic therapy:** Antiandrogens have been used to treat hypersexual paraphilias in men.

Biological sex is one's physiological sex as determined by genetic or anatomic factors. *Gender identity* is one's internal, subjective feeling of being either male or female and usually develops by age 3.

▶ GENDER IDENTITY DISORDER

Gender identity disorder is commonly referred to as *transsexuality*. People with this disorder have the subjective feeling that they were born the wrong sex. They may dress as the opposite sex, take sex hormones, or undergo sex change operations.

Gender identity disorder is more common in men than women. It is associated with an increased incidence of major depression, anxiety disorders, and suicide.

▶ HOMOSEXUALITY

Homosexuality is a sexual or romantic desire for people of the same sex. It is a normal variant of sexual orientation. It occurs in 3 to 10% of men and 1 to 5% of women. The etiology of homosexuality is unknown, but genetic or prenatal factors may play a role.

Distress about one's sexual orientation is considered a dysfunction that should be treated with individual psychotherapy and/or group therapy.

Psychotherapies

► PSYCHOANALYSIS AND RELATED THERAPIES

Psychoanalysis and its related therapies are derived from Sigmund Freud's psychoanalytic theories of the mind. Freud proposed that behaviors result from *unconscious* mental processes, including defense mechanisms and conflicts between one's ego, id, superego, and external reality. Since the time of Freud, many other psychoanalytic theories have been developed. Influential theorists have included Melanie Klein, Heinz Kohut, Michael Blaint, Margaret Mahler, and others.

Examples of psychoanalytic therapies include:

- Psychoanalysis
- Psychoanalytically oriented psychotherapy
- Brief dynamic therapy
- Interpersonal therapy

► FREUD'S THEORIES OF THE MIND

Topographic Theories

1. *Unconscious*—includes repressed thoughts that are out of one's awareness; involves *primary process* thinking (primitive, pleasure-seeking urges with no regard to logic or time, prominent in children and psychotics)
2. *Preconscious*—contains memories that are easy to bring into awareness
3. *Conscious*—involves current thoughts and secondary process thinking (logical, mature, and can delay gratification)

Structural Theories

1. *Id*—unconscious; involves instinctual sexual/aggressive urges and primary process thinking
2. *Ego*—serves as a mediator between the id and external environment and seeks to develop satisfying interpersonal relationships; uses *defense mechanisms* (see below) to control instinctual urges and distinguishes

Normal development:
- Id present at birth
- Ego present after birth
- Superego present by age 6

fantasy from reality using *reality testing*. Problems with reality testing occur in psychotic individuals.

3. *Superego*—moral conscience

Defense mechanisms are used by the ego to protect oneself and relieve anxiety by keeping conflicts out of awareness. They are *unconscious* processes that are normal and healthy when used in moderation. However, excessive use of certain defense mechanisms may be seen in some psychiatric disorders.

Defense mechanisms are often classified hierarchically. *Mature* defense mechanisms are healthy and adaptive, and they are seen in normal adults. *Neurotic* defenses are encountered in obsessive–compulsive patients, hysterical patients, and adults under stress. *Immature* defenses are seen in children, adolescents, psychotic patients, and some nonpsychotic patients. They are the most primitive defense mechanisms.

Mature Defenses

1. **Altruism**—performing acts that benefit others in order to vicariously experience pleasure
2. **Humor**—expressing feelings through comedy without causing discomfort to self or others
3. **Sublimation**— satisfying socially objectionable impulses in an acceptable manner (thus *channeling* them rather than *preventing* them) (*Clinical example:* Person with unconscious urges to physically control others becomes a prison guard.)
4. **Suppression**—purposely ignoring an unacceptable impulse or emotion in order to diminish discomfort and accomplish a task (*Clinical example:* Nurse who feels nauseated by an infected wound puts aside feelings of disgust to clean wound and provide necessary patient care.)

Neurotic Defenses

1. **Controlling**—regulating situations and events of external environment to relieve anxiety
2. **Displacement**—shifting emotions from an undesirable situation to one that is personally tolerable (*Clinical example:* Student who is angry at his mother talks back to his teacher the next day and refuses to obey her instructions.)
3. **Intellectualization**—avoiding negative feelings by excessive use of intellectual functions and by focusing on irrelevant details or inanimate objects (*Clinical example:* Physician dying from colon cancer describes the pathophysiology of his disease in detail to his 12-year-old son.)
4. **Isolation of affect**—unconsciously limiting the experience of feelings or emotions associated with a stressful life event in order to avoid anxiety (*Clinical example:* Woman describes the recent death of her beloved husband without emotion.)
5. **Rationalization**—creating explanations of an event in order to justify outcomes or behaviors and to make them acceptable. (*Clinical example:*

"My boss fired me today because she's short-tempered and impulsive, not because I haven't done a good job.")

6. **Reaction formation**—doing the opposite of an unacceptable impulse (*Clinical example:* Man who is in love with his coworker insults her.)

7. **Repression**—preventing a thought or feeling from entering consciousness (Repression is unconscious, whereas suppression is a conscious act.)

Immature Defenses

1. **Acting out**—giving in to an impulse, even if socially inappropriate, in order to avoid the anxiety of suppressing that impulse (*Clinical example:* Man who has been told his therapist is going on vacation "forgets" his last appointment and skips it.)

2. **Denial**—not accepting reality that is too painful (*Clinical example:* Woman who has been scheduled for a breast mass biopsy cancels her appointment because she believes she is healthy.)

3. **Regression**—performing behaviors from an earlier stage of development in order to avoid tension associated with current phase of development (*Clinical example:* Woman brings her childhood teddy bear to the hospital when she has to spend the night.)

4. **Projection**—attributing objectionable thoughts or emotions to others (*Clinical example:* Husband who is attracted to other women believes his wife is having an affair.)

Other Defense Mechanisms

1. **Splitting**—labeling people as all good or all bad (often seen in borderline personality disorder) (*Clinical example:* Woman who tells her doctor, "you and the nurses are the only people who understand me; all the other doctors are mean and impatient.")

2. **Undoing**—attempting to reverse a situation by adopting a new behavior (*Clinical example:* Man who has had a brief fantasy of killing his wife by sabotaging her car takes the car in for a complete checkup.)

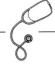

Beware when your patient thinks you're so cool to talk to but hates the evil attending. That's splitting. Impress your attending and point it out.

The goal of psychoanalysis is to resolve *unconscious conflicts* by bringing repressed experiences and feelings into awareness and integrating them into the patient's personality. Psychoanalysis is therefore *insight oriented*. Patients best suited for psychoanalysis have the following characteristics: Under age 40, not psychotic, intelligent, and stable in relationships and daily living.

Psychoanalysis may be useful in the treatment of:
- Personality disorders
- Anxiety disorders
- Obsessive–compulsive disorder
- Problems coping with life events
- Anorexia nervosa
- Sexual disorders
- Dysthymic disorder

During treatment, the patient usually lies on a couch with the therapist seated out of view. Patients attend sessions four to five times a week for multiple years.

Important Concepts and Techniques Used in Psychoanalysis

Free association: the patient is asked to say whatever comes into his or her mind during therapy sessions. The purpose is to bring forth thoughts and feelings from the unconscious so that the therapist may interpret them.

Dream interpretation: Dreams are seen to represent conflict between urges and fears. Interpretation of dreams by the psychoanalyst is used to help achieve therapeutic goals.

Therapeutic alliance: This is the bond between the therapist and the patient, who work together toward a therapeutic goal.

Transference: Projection of unconscious feelings about important figures in the patient's life onto the therapist. Interpretation of transference is used to help the patient gain insight and resolve unconscious conflict. (*Example:* Patient who has repressed feelings of abandonment by her father becomes angry when her therapist is 5 minutes late for an appointment.)

Countertransference: Projection of unconscious feelings about important figures in the therapist's life onto the patient. The therapist must remain aware of countertransference issues, as they may interfere with his or her objectivity.

Psychoanalysis-Related Therapies

Examples of psychoanalysis-related therapies include:

1. *Psychoanalytically oriented psychotherapy* and *brief dynamic psychotherapy:* These employ similar techniques and theories as psychoanalysis, but they are briefer (weekly sessions for 6 months to 1½ years) and involve face-to-face sessions between the therapist and patient (no couch).

2. *Interpersonal therapy:* Focuses on development of social skills to help treat certain psychiatric disorders. Treatment is short (weekly sessions for 3 to 6 months). Idea is to improve interpersonal relations.

3. *Supportive psychotherapy:* Purpose is to help patient feel safe during a difficult time. Treatment is not insight oriented but instead focuses on empathy, understanding, and education. Supportive therapy is commonly used as adjunctive treatment in even the most severe mental disorders. Helps to build up the patient's healthy defenses. Dependency is encouraged.

▶ BEHAVIORAL THERAPY

Behavioral therapy seeks to treat psychiatric disorders by helping patients change behaviors that contribute to their symptoms. It can be used to extinguish maladaptive behaviors (such as phobias, sexual dysfunction, compulsions, etc.) by replacing them with healthy alternatives.

Learning Theory

Behavioral therapy is based on **learning theory,** which states that behaviors can be learned by *conditioning* and can similarly be unlearned by *deconditioning*.

Conditioning

Classical conditioning: A stimulus can eventually evoke a conditioned response. (*Example*: Pavlov's dog would salivate when hearing a bell because the dog had learned that bells were always followed by food.)

Operant conditioning: Behaviors can be learned when followed by positive or negative *reinforcement*. (*Example*: Skinner's box—a rat happened upon a lever and received food; eventually it learned to press the lever for food [trial-and-error learning].)

Behavioral Therapy Techniques (Deconditioning)

Systemic desensitization: The patient performs relaxation techniques while being exposed to increasing doses of an anxiety-provoking stimulus. Gradually, he or she learns to associate the stimulus with a state of relaxation. Commonly used to treat phobic disorders. (*Example*: A patient who has a fear of spiders is first shown a photograph of a spider, followed by a stuffed animal, a videotape, and finally a live spider.)

Flooding and implosion: Through habituation, the patient is confronted with a real (flooding) or imagined (implosion) anxiety-provoking stimulus and not allowed to withdraw from it until he or she feels calm and in control. Relaxation exercises are used to help the patient tolerate the stimulus. Commonly used to treat phobic disorders. (*Example*: A patient who has a fear of flying is made to fly in an airplane [flooding] or imagine flying [implosion].)

Aversion therapy: A negative stimulus (such as an electric shock) is repeatedly paired with a specific behavior to create an unpleasant response. Commonly used to treat addictions or paraphilias. (*Example*: An alcoholic patient is prescribed Antabuse, which makes him ill every time he drinks alcohol.)

Token economy: Rewards are given after specific behaviors to positively reinforce them. Commonly used to encourage showering, shaving, and other positive behaviors in disorganized or mentally retarded individuals.

Biofeedback: Physiological data (such as heart rate or blood pressure measurements) are given to patients as they try to mentally control physiological states. Commonly used to treat migraines, hypertension, chronic pain, asthma, and incontinence. (*Example*: A patient is given her heart rate and blood pressure measurements during a migraine while being instructed to mentally control visceral changes that affect her pain.)

▶ COGNITIVE THERAPY

Cognitive therapy seeks to correct faulty assumptions and negative feelings that exacerbate psychiatric symptoms. The patient is taught to identify maladaptive thoughts and replace them with positive ones. Most commonly used to treat depressive and anxiety disorders. May also be used for paranoid personality disorder, obsessive–compulsive disorder, somatoform disorders, and eating disorders. Cognitive therapy can be more effective than medication.

Clinical Example of the Cognitive Theory of Depression

Faulty assumptions: If I were smart I would do well on tests. I must not be smart since I received average grades this semester.

Faulty assumptions lead to:
Negative thoughts: I am stupid. I will never amount to anything worthwhile. Nobody likes a worthless person.

Negative thoughts then lead to:
Psychopathology: Depression

Three or more patients with a similar problem or pathology meet together with a therapist for group sessions. Any of the psychotherapeutic techniques may be employed, including psychoanalytical, behavioral, cognitive, educational, and so on.

Certain groups are *leaderless* (including 12-step groups like Alcoholics Anonymous) and do not have a therapist present to facilitate the group. These groups meet to discuss problems, share feelings, and provide support to each other.

Group therapy is especially useful in the treatment of substance abuse, adjustment disorders, and personality disorders. Advantages of group therapy over individual therapy include:

- Patients get immediate feedback from their peers.
- Patients may gain insight into their own condition by listening to others with similar problems.
- If a therapist is present, there is an opportunity to observe interactions between others who may be eliciting a variety of transferences.

Family therapy is useful as an adjunctive treatment in many psychiatric conditions because:

1. A person's problems usually affect the entire family. He or she may be viewed differently and treated differently after the development of psychopathology, and new tensions and conflicts within the family may arise.
2. Psychopathology may arise partly or entirely from dysfunction within the family unit. These conditions are most effectively treated with the entire family present.

The goals of family therapy are to reduce conflict, help members understand each other's needs (*mutual accommodation*), and help the unit cope with internally destructive forces. **Boundaries** between family members may be too rigid or too permeable, and **"triangles"** may result when two family members form an alliance against a third member. The therapist may assist in correcting these problems as well. (*Example of boundaries that may be too permeable:*

Mother and daughter smoke marijuana together and share intimate details about their sexual activities.)

▶ MARITAL THERAPY

Marital therapy is useful in the treatment of conflicts, sexual problems, and communication problems. Usually, the therapist sees the couple together **(conjoint therapy)**, but they may be seen separately **(concurrent therapy)**. In addition, each person may have a separate therapist and be seen individually **(collaborative therapy)**. In the treatment of sexual problems, two therapists may each see the couple together **(four-way therapy)**. Relative contraindications include lack of motivation by one or both spouses and severe illness in one of the spouses, such as psychosis.

DIALECTICAL BEHAVIORAL THERAPY

Developed by Marsha Linehan, effectiveness demonstrated in research control study.

- Specific treatment for borderline personality disorder
- Teaches coping skills with both individual and group therapy
- 1- to 2-year commitment required; treatment usually 2 to 3 times per week
- Solution-focused therapy
- Main goals:
  1. Reduce self-injurious behaviors
  2. Decrease hospitalizations
- Key topics patient is taught to use in everyday life:
  1. Mindfulness
  2. Interpersonal effectiveness
  3. Emotion regulation
  4. Distress tolerance

Psychopharmacology

The major categories of antidepressants are:
- Tricyclic antidepressants (TCAs)
- Monoamine oxidase inhibitors (MAOIs)
- Selective serotonin reuptake inhibitors (SSRIs)
- Atypical antidepressants

All antidepressants are considered equally effective in treating major depression but differ in safety and side effect profiles. About 70% of patients with major depression will respond to antidepressant medication. Antidepressants have **no abuse potential** and do not *elevate* mood.

Because of their safety and tolerability, SSRIs and atypical antidepressants have become the most common agents used to treat major depression. However, the choice of a particular medication used for a given patient should be made based on:
- Patient's symptoms
- Previous treatment responses by the patient or a family member to a particular drug
- Medication side effect profile
- Comorbid conditions
- Risk of suicide

Sympathomimetics (amphetamine-based drugs) may be effective in patients who cannot tolerate or do not respond to traditional antidepressant medications. However, they are used only rarely due to their addiction potential. Use should be short term and carefully monitored.

OTHER DISORDERS FOR WHICH ANTIDEPRESSANTS ARE USED

Obsessive–compulsive disorder (OCD): SSRIs, TCAs
Panic disorder: SSRIs, TCAs, MAOIs
Eating disorders: SSRIs, TCAs, and MAOIs
Dysthymia: SSRIs
Social phobia: MAOIs and SSRIs
Posttraumatic stress disorder: SSRIs, TCAs
Irritable bowel syndrome: SSRIs, TCAs
Enuresis: TCAs
Neuropathic pain: TCAs
Migraine headaches: TCAs, SSRIs, bupropion
Smoking cessation: Bupropion
Autism: SSRIs
Premenstrual dysphoric disorder: SSRIs
Depressive phase of manic depression: SSRIs, bupropion
Insomnia: Mirtazapine, TCAs

The hallmark of TCA toxicity is a widened QRS (>100 msec), used as threshold to treatment.

The mainstay of treatment for TCA overdose is IV sodium bicarbonate.

TCA side effects:
Anti-HAM (histamine, adrenergic, muscarinic)

Tricyclic Antidepressants (TCAs)

TCAs inhibit the reuptake of norepinephrine and serotonin, increasing availability in the synapse. They are rarely used as first-line agents because they have a higher incidence of side effects, require greater monitoring of dosing, and can be **lethal in overdose.**

Patients are usually started on low doses to allow acclimation to the common early anticholinergic side effects before achieving therapeutic doses. Examples of TCAs include:

- **Imipramine (Tofranil)**
- **Amitriptyline (Elavil)**
- **Trimipramine (Surmontil)**
- **Nortriptyline (Pamelor)**—least likely to cause orthostatic hypotension
- **Desipramine (Norpramin)**—least sedating, least anticholinergic side effects
- **Clomipramine (Anafranil)**—most serotonin specific, useful in treatment of OCD
- **Doxepin (Sinequan)**

SIDE EFFECTS

The side effects of TCAs are mostly due to their lack of specificity and interaction with other receptors.

1. Antihistaminic properties: Sedation
2. Antiadrenergic properties (cardiovascular side effects): Orthostatic hypotension (most life threatening), tachycardia, arrhythmias
3. Antimuscarinic effects: Dry mouth, constipation, urinary retention, blurred vision, tachycardia
4. Weight gain
5. **Lethal in overdose**—must assess suicide risk!! A 1-week supply of these drugs can be lethal in overdose.
6. Major complications—3Cs: Convulsions, coma, cardiotoxicity. Avoid in patients with preexisting conduction abnormalities.

Monoamine Oxidase Inhibitors (MAOIs)

MAOIs prevent the inactivation of biogenic amines such as *norepinephrine, serotonin, dopamine,* and *tyramine* (an intermediate in the conversion of tyrosine to norepinephrine). By irreversibly inhibiting the enzymes *MAO-A* and *-B*, MAOIs increase the amount of these transmitters available in synapses. MAO-A preferentially deactivates serotonin, and MAO-B preferentially deactivates norepinephrine/epinephrine. *Both* types also act on dopamine and tyramine.

MAOIs are not used as first-line agents because of the increased safety and tolerability of newer agents. However, MAOIs are considered very effective for certain types of **refractory depression** and in refractory panic disorder.

Examples: Phenelzine (Nardil), tranylcypromine (Parnate), isocarboxazid (Marplan)

SIDE EFFECTS

- *Common side effects:* Orthostatic hypotension, drowsiness, weight gain, sexual dysfunction, dry mouth, sleep dysfunction

- *Serotonin syndrome* occurs when **SSRIs** and **MAOIs** are taken together. Initially characterized by lethargy, restlessness, confusion, flushing, diaphoresis, tremor, and myoclonic jerks. May progress to hyperthermia, hypertonicity, rhabdomyolysis, renal failure, convulsions, coma, and death. Wait at least 2 weeks before switching from SSRI to MAOI.
- *Hypertensive crisis:* Risk when MAOIs are taken with **tyramine**-rich foods or **sympathomimetics.** Foods with tyramine (red Chianti wine, cheese, chicken liver, fava beans, cured meats) cause a buildup of stored catecholamines.

First step when suspecting serotonin syndrome: Discontinue medication

Selective Serotonin Reuptake Inhibitors (SSRIs)

SSRIs inhibit presynaptic serotonin pumps, leading to increased availability of serotonin in synaptic clefts. SSRIs all have similar efficacy and side effects despite structural differences. They are the most commonly prescribed antidepressants due to several distinct advantages:
- Low incidence of side effects
- No food restrictions
- Much safer in overdose

Sympathomimetics may be found in over-the-counter cold remedies.

SSRIs are also used in the treatment of some anxiety disorders, OCD, and premenstrual dysphoric disorder.

Examples of SSRIs include:
- **Fluoxetine (Prozac)**—longest half-life with active metabolites: Do not need to taper
- **Sertraline (Zoloft)**—highest risk for gastrointestinal (GI) disturbances
- **Paroxetine (Paxil)**—most serotonin specific, most activating (stimulant)
- **Fluvoxamine (Luvox)**—currently approved only for use in OCD
- **Citalopram (Celexa)**—used in Europe for 12 years prior to FDA approval in the United States
- **Escitalopram (Lexapro)**—levo enantiomer of citalopram; similar efficacy, fewer side effects, much more expensive

SIDE EFFECTS

SSRIs have significantly fewer side effects than TCAs and MAOIs due to serotonin selectivity (they do not act on histamine, adrenergic, or muscarinic receptors).

Side effects of SSRIs include:
- Sexual dysfunction (25 to 30%)
- GI disturbance
- Insomnia
- Headache
- Anorexia, weight loss
- Serotonin syndrome when used with MAOIs (see above)

Atypical Antidepressants

Include serotonin/norepinephrine reuptake inhibitors (**SNRIs**), norepinephrine/dopamine reuptake inhibitors (**NDRIs**), serotonin antagonist and reuptake inhibitors (**SARIs**), and norepinephrine and serotonin antagonists (**NASAs**)

SNRIs

Venlafaxine (Effexor): Venlafaxine is especially useful in treating refractory depression and CAP. It has a very low drug interaction potential. Side effect profiles similar to SSRIs (see above). In addition, venlafaxine can increase BP; do not use in patients with untreated or labile BP. Potential withdrawal symptoms can be seen with 1–3 missed doses; not life threatening, but very uncomfortable (including flulike symptoms and electric-like shocks or zaps).

NDRIs

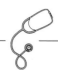

Bupropion can lower seizure threshold. Use with caution in epileptics.

Bupropion (Wellbutrin): Bupropion is commonly used to aid in smoking cessation, and it is also useful in the treatment of seasonal affective disorder and adult attention deficit hyperactivity disorder (ADHD). Its most significant advantage is its relative **lack of sexual side effects** as compared to the SSRIs. Bupropion's dopaminergic effect in higher doses can exacerbate psychosis. Side effects are similar to SSRIs, with increased sweating and increased risk of **seizures** and **psychosis** at high doses. They are not optimal for patients with significant anxiety and are contraindicated in patients with seizure or active eating disorders and in those currently on an MAOI.

SARIs

Trazodone causes priapism: t**RAZ**odone will **RAISE** the bone.

Nefazodone (Serzone) and trazodone (Desyrel): These are especially useful in treatment of refractory major depression, major depression with anxiety, and **insomnia** (secondary to its sedative effects). Side effects include nausea, dizziness, orthostatic hypotension, cardiac arrhythmias, **sedation,** and **priapism** (sedation and priapism especially with **trazodone**).

NASAs

Mirtazapine (Remeron): Useful in the treatment of refractory major depression, especially in patients who need to gain weight. Side effects include sedation, **weight gain,** dizziness, somnolence, tremor, and agranulocytosis. Maximal sedative effect at doses of 15 mg and less; at higher doses, it increases norepinephrine upake and is therefore less sedating.

▶ ANTIPSYCHOTICS

Antipsychotics are used to treat psychotic disorders and psychotic symptoms associated with other psychiatric and medical illnesses. *Traditional* antipsychotics are classified according to potency and work by blocking dopamine receptors. *Atypical* (newer) antipsychotics block both dopamine and serotonin receptors; however, their effect on dopamine is weaker, so they are associated with fewer side effects.

Traditional Antipsychotics

Low potency: Have a lower affinity for dopamine receptors and therefore a higher dose is required. Remember, *potency* refers to the action on dopamine receptors, not the level of efficacy.

- Chlorpromazine (Thorazine)
- Thioridazine (Mellaril)

These antipsychotics have a higher incidence of anticholinergic and antihistaminic side effects than high-potency traditional antipsychotics. They have a lower incidence of extrapyramidal side effects (EPSEs) and neuroleptic malignant syndrome. (See below for detailed description of side effects.)

High potency: Have greater affinity for dopamine receptors, and therefore a relatively low dose is needed to achieve effect.
- Haloperidol (Haldol)
- Fluphenazine (Prolixin)
- Trifluoperazine (Stelazine)
- Perphenazine (Trilafon)
- Pimozide (Orap)

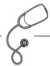

Haloperidol and fluphenazine are also available in long-acting forms (decanoate)—administer IM every 2 to 3 weeks for fluphenazine and 4 to 5 weeks for haloperidol.

These antipsychotics have a higher incidence of **EPSEs** and neuroleptic malignant syndrome than low-potency traditional antipsychotics (see below). They have a lower incidence of anticholinergic and antihistaminic side effects.

Both traditional and atypical neuroleptics have similar efficacies in treating the presence of *positive psychotic symptoms*, such as hallucinations and delusions; atypical antipsychotics have been shown to be more effective in treating *negative symptoms* (such as flattened affect and social withdrawal).

Side Effects of Traditional Antipsychotics

Side effects and sequelae of traditional antipsychotics include:

1. **Antidopaminergic effects:**
   - **Extrapyramidal side effects**
     - *Parkinsonism*—masklike face, cogwheel rigidity, pill-rolling tremor.
     - *Akathisia*—subjective anxiety and restlessness, objective fidgetiness
     - *Dystonia*—sustained contraction of muscles of neck, tongue, eyes (painful)
   - *Hyperprolactinemia*—leading to decreased libido, galactorrhea, gynecomastia, impotence, amenorrhea, osteoporosis

Dopamine normally inhibits prolactin and acetylcholine secretion.

Treatment of EPSEs includes reducing dose of antipsychotic and administering antiparkinsonian, anticholinergic, or antihistaminic medications, such as amantadine (Symmetrel), Benadryl, or benztropine (Cogentin).

2. **Anti-HAM effects:** Caused by actions on **h**istaminic, **a**drenergic, and **m**uscarinic receptors:
   - *Antihistaminic*—results in sedation
   - *Anti–alpha adrenergic*—results in orthostatic hypotension, cardiac abnormalities, and sexual dysfunction
   - *Antimuscarinic*—anticholinergic effects: Dry mouth, tachycardia, urinary retention, blurry vision, constipation
3. **Weight gain**
4. Elevated **liver** enzymes, jaundice
5. Ophthalmologic problems (irreversible retinal pigmentation with high doses of Mellaril, deposits in lens and cornea with chlorpromazine)
6. **Dermatologic** problems, including rashes and photosensitivity (blue-gray skin discoloration with chlorpromazine)
7. **Seizures:** Antipsychotics lower seizure thresholds. Low-potency antipsychotics are more likely to cause seizures than high potency.

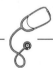

Tardive dyskinesia hypothesized to be caused by increase in number of dopamine receptors, causing lower levels of acetylcholine.

Young man admitted to hospital and put on antipsychotic becomes catatonic and will not get out of bed. Next step: Stop medications.

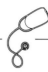

8. **Tardive dyskinesia:** Choreoathetoid (writhing) movements of mouth and tongue that may occur in patients who have used neuroleptics for more than 6 months. It most often occurs in older women. Though 50% of cases will spontaneously remit, untreated cases may be *permanent.*

Treatment involves discontinuation of current antipsychotic if clinically possible (and sometimes administration of anxiolytics or cholinomimetics).

9. **Neuroleptic malignant syndrome:** Though rare, occurs most often in males early in treatment with neuroleptics. It is a **medical emergency** and has a 20% mortality rate if left untreated. It is often preceded by a catatonic state. It is characterized by:
   Fever (most common presenting symptom)
   Autonomic instability (tachycardia, labile hypertension, diaphoresis)
   Leukocytosis
   Tremor
   Elevated creatine phosphokinase (CPK)
   Rigidity (*lead pipe* rigidity is considered almost universal)

Treatment involves discontinuation of current medications and administration of supportive medical care (hydration, cooling, etc.). Sodium dantrolene, bromocriptine, and amantadine are also useful but are infrequently used because of their own side effects. This is *not* an allergic reaction. Patient is not prevented from restarting the same neuroleptic at a later time.

Atypical Antipsychotics

Atypical antipsychotics block both dopamine and serotonin receptors and are associated with **fewer side effects** than traditional antipsychotics; in particular, they rarely cause EPSEs, tardive dyskinesia, or neuroleptic malignant syndrome. They are more effective in treating **negative symptoms** of schizophrenia than traditional antipsychotics. Because they have fewer side effects and increased effectiveness in treating negative symptoms, these drugs are now first line in the treatment of schizophrenia.

EXAMPLES

Atypical antipsychotics include:
- Clozapine (Clozaril)
- Risperidone (Risperdal)
- Quetiapine (Seroquel)
- Olanzapine (Zyprexa)
- Ziprasidone (Geodon)

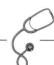

Quetiapine and ziprasidone both have FDA approval for treatment of mania.

SIDE EFFECTS

- Some anti-HAM effects (antihistaminic, antiadrenergic, and antimuscarinic)
- 1% incidence of agranulocytosis and 2 to 5% incidence of seizures with clozapine
- Olanzapine can cause hyperlipidemia, glucose intolerance, weight gain, and liver toxicity; monitor liver function tests (LFTs).
- Quetiapine has less propensity for weight gain but has been shown to cause cataracts in beagle dogs, so periodic (every 6 months) slit lamp examination is recommended.

Patients on clozapine must have weekly blood draws to check white blood cell counts because it can cause agranulocytosis.

Mood stabilizers are also known as *antimanics* and are used to treat acute mania and to help prevent relapses of manic episodes. Less commonly, they may be used for:

- Potentiation of antidepressants in patients with major depression refractory to monotherapy
- Potentiation of antipsychotics in patients with schizophrenia
- Enhancement of abstinence in treatment of alcoholism
- Treatment of aggression and impulsivity (dementia, intoxication, mental retardation, personality disorders, general medical conditions)

Mood stabilizers include lithium and two anticonvulsants, carbamazepine and valproic acid.

> **Antipsychotics may be used as adjuncts to mood stabilizers for behavioral control early in the course of a manic episode if psychotic symptoms are present.**

Lithium

Lithium is the drug of choice in the treatment of acute mania and as prophylaxis for both manic and depressive episodes in bipolar disorder. Its exact mechanism of action is unknown, but it has been shown to alter neuronal sodium transport. (Lithium is in the same column as sodium in the periodic table.)

Lithium is secreted by the kidney, and its onset of action takes 5 to 7 days. Blood levels correlate with clinical efficacy. The major drawback of lithium is its high incidence of side effects and very narrow therapeutic index:

- Therapeutic range: 0.7 to 1.2 (Individual patients can become toxic even within this range.)
- Toxic: > 1.5
- Lethal: > 2.0

> **Factors that affect Li+ levels:**
> - NSAIDs ($\downarrow$)
> - Aspirin
> - Dehydration ($\uparrow$)
> - Salt deprivation ($\uparrow$)
> - Impaired renal function ($\uparrow$)
> - Diuretics

SIDE EFFECTS

Side effects of lithium include fine tremor, sedation, ataxia, thirst, metallic taste, polyuria, edema, weight gain, GI problems, benign leukocytosis, thyroid enlargement, **hypothyroidism,** and **nephrogenic diabetes insipidus.**

Toxic levels of lithium cause altered mental status, coarse tremors, convulsions, and death. Clinicians need to regularly monitor blood levels of lithium, thyroid function (thyroid-stimulating hormone), and kidney function (glomerular filtration rate).

Carbamazepine (Tegretol)

Carbamazepine is an anticonvulsant that is especially useful in treating *mixed* episodes and *rapid-cycling* bipolar disorder. It is also used in the management of trigeminal neuralgia. It acts by blocking sodium channels and inhibiting action potentials. Its onset of action is 5 to 7 days.

SIDE EFFECTS

Side effects include skin rash, drowsiness, ataxia, slurred speech, **leukopenia, hyponatremia, aplastic anemia,** and **agranulocytosis.** It elevates liver enzymes and has teratogenic effects when used during pregnancy **(neural tube defects).** Pretreatment complete blood count (CBC) and LFTs must be obtained and monitored regularly.

Valproic Acid (Depakene)

Valproic acid is an anticonvulsant that is especially useful in treating mixed manic episodes and rapid-cycling bipolar disorder. Its mechanism of action is unknown, but it has been shown to increase central nervous system (CNS) levels of gamma-aminobutyric acid (GABA).

SIDE EFFECTS

Side effects include sedation, weight gain, alopecia, hemorrhagic pancreatitis, **hepatotoxicity,** and **thrombocytopenia.** It has teratogenic effects during pregnancy **(neural tube defects).** Monitoring of LFTs and CBCs is necessary.

> ▶ **ANXIOLYTICS/HYPNOTICS**

Anxiolytics, including benzodiazepines, barbiturates, and buspirone, are the most widely prescribed psychotropic medications. In general, they all work by diffusely depressing the CNS, causing a sedative effect. Common indications for anxiolytics/hypnotics include:

- Anxiety disorders
- Muscle spasm
- Seizures
- Sleep disorders
- Alcohol withdrawal
- Anesthesia induction

BDZs can be lethal when mixed with alcohol.

Benzodiazepines (BDZs)

Benzodiazepines are first-line anxiolytics. Advantages include safety at high doses (as opposed to barbiturates). A significant limitation is imposed on the duration of BDZ use due to their potential for tolerance and dependence after prolonged use. Benzodiazepines work by potentiating the effects of GABA.

EXAMPLES OF BDZs

Long Acting (1 to 3 Days)
Chlordiazepoxide (Librium)—used in alcohol detoxification, presurgery anxiety
Diazepam (Valium)—rapid onset, used in treatment of anxiety and seizure control
Flurazepam (Dalmane)—rapid onset, treatment of insomnia

Intermediate Acting (10 to 20 Hours)
Alprazolam (Xanax)—treatment of panic attacks
Clonazepam (Klonopin)—treatment of panic attacks, anxiety
Lorazepam (Ativan)—treatment of panic attacks, alcohol withdrawal
Temazepam (Restoril)—treatment of insomnia

Short Acting (3 to 8 Hours)
Oxazepam (Serax)
Triazolam (Halcion)—rapid onset, treatment of insomnia

Drowsiness, impairment of intellectual function, reduced motor coordination. *Toxicity*: Respiratory depression in overdose, especially when combined with alcohol

Zolpidem (Ambien)/Zaleplon (Sonata)

- Used for short-term treatment of insomnia
- Selectively bind to benzodiazepine binding site on GABA receptor
- No anticonvulsant or muscle relaxant properties
- No withdrawal effects
- Minimal rebound insomnia
- Little or no tolerance/dependence occurs with prolonged use
- Sonata—newer, has shorter half-life than Ambien
- Chemically not a BDZ, although same effect

Buspirone (BuSpar)

- Alternative to BDZ or venlafaxine for treating generalized anxiety disorder
- Slower onset of action than benzodiazepines (takes 1 to 2 weeks for effect)
- Anxiolytic action is at 5HT-1A receptor (partial agonist)
- Does not potentiate the CNS depression of alcohol (useful in alcoholics)
- Low potential for abuse/addiction

Propranolol

This beta blocker is particularly useful in treating the autonomic effects of panic attacks or performance anxiety, such as palpitations, sweating, and tachycardia. It can also be used to treat akathisia (side effect of typical antipsychotics).

▶ **SIDE EFFECTS IN A NUTSHELL**

Most important facts to know for exam:

HAM side effects (*antihistamine*—*sedation*; *antiadrenergic*—*hypotension*; *antimuscarinic*—dry mouth, blurred vision, urinary retention)
- Found in **TCAs** and **low-potency antipsychotics**

Serotonin syndrome: Confusion, flushing, diaphoresis, tremor, myoclonic jerks, hyperthermia, hypertonicity, rhabdomyolysis, renal failure, and death
- Occurs when **SSRIs and MAOIs are combined**
- Treatment: Stop drugs

Hypertensive crisis: Caused by a buildup of stored catecholamines
- **MAOIs** plus **foods with tyramine** (red wine, cheese, chicken liver, cured meats) or plus **sympathomimetics**

Extrapyramidal side effects
- *Parkinsonism*—masklike face, cogwheel rigity, pill-rolling tremor
- *Akathisia*—restlessness and *agitation*

- *Dystonia—sustained contraction of muscles* of neck, tongue, eyes
  - Occurs with **high-potency** traditional antipsychotics
  - **Reversible,** occurs within days
  - **Can be life threatening** (*example*—dystonia of the diaphragm causing asphyxiation)

Hyperprolactinemia
- Occurs with **high-potency** traditional antipsychotics

Tardive dyskinesia: Choreoathetoid muscle movements, usually of mouth and tongue. More likely in women than men
- Occurs after years of antipsychotic use (particularly high-potency typical antipsychotics); can be **irreversible**
- Patients on antipsychotics should be monitored for this with various screening exams (abnormal involuntary movement scale [AIMS], DISCUS) every 6 months.

Neuroleptic malignant syndrome: Fever, tachycardia, hypertension, tremor, elevated CPK, "lead pipe" rigidity
- Can be caused by all antipsychotics after short or long time (increased with high-potency traditional antipsychotics)
- A **medical emergency** with 20% mortality rate

► **SUMMARY OF MEDICATIONS THAT MAY CAUSE PSYCHIATRIC SYMPTOMS**

Psychosis

May be caused by sympathomimetics, analgesics, antibiotics (such as isoniazid), anticholinergics, anticonvulsants, antihistamines, corticosteroids, and antiparkinsonian agents

Agitation/Confusion/Delirium

May be caused by antipsychotics, antidepressants, antiarrhythmics, antineoplastics, corticosteroids, cardiac glycosides, NSAIDs, antiasthmatics, antibiotics, antihypertensives, antiparkinsonian agents, and thyroid hormones

Depression

May be caused by antihypertensives, antiparkinsonian agents, corticosteroids, calcium channel blockers, NSAIDs, antibiotics, and peptic ulcer drugs

Anxiety

May be caused by sympathomimetics, antiasthmatics, antiparkinsonian agents, hypoglycemics, NSAIDs, and thyroid hormones

Sedation/Poor Concentration

May be caused by antianxiety agents/hypnotics, anticholinergics, antibiotics, and antihistamines

Legal Issues in Psychiatry

▶ CONFIDENTIALITY

All information regarding a doctor–patient relationship should be held confidential except in the following situations:

1. When sharing relevant information with other staff members who are also treating the patient
2. If subpoenaed—physician must supply all requested information
3. If child abuse is suspected—obligated to report to the proper authorities
4. If patient is an immediate danger to others—obligated to report to the proper authorities (Tarasoff Duty)
5. If a patient is suicidal—physician may need to admit the patient, with or without the patient's consent, and share information with the hospital staff.

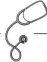

The obligation of a physician to report patients who are potentially harmful to others is called the *Tarasoff Duty,* based on a legal case.

▶ ADMISSION TO A PSYCHIATRIC HOSPITAL

The two main categories of admission to a psychiatric hospital are:

1. *Voluntary admission:* Patient requests or agrees to be admitted to the psychiatric ward. The patient is first examined by a staff psychiatrist, who determines if he or she should be hospitalized.
2. *Involuntary admission* (also known as *civil commitment*): Patient is found by two staff physicians to be potentially harmful to self or others (suicidal, homicidal, unable to care for self, etc.), so may be hospitalized against his or her will for a certain number of days (depending on laws of state). After the set number of days have passed, the case must be reviewed by an independent board to determine if continued hospitalization is necessary. Patients must always be provided with a copy of the commitment (or "hold") papers, have their rights explained to them, and must have any questions answered pertaining to the commitment.

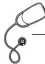

Patients who are admitted against their will retain legal rights and can contest their admission in court at any time.

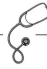

Parens patriae is the legal doctrine that allows civil commitment for citizens unable to care for themselves.

Elements of informed consent: NARCC
- **N**ame/purpose of treatment
- **A**lternatives
- **R**isks/benefits
- **C**onsequences of refusing
- **C**apacity (patient must have)

Informed consent for treatment of minors is not required from parents in:
- Obstetric care
- Treatment of STDs
- Treatment of substance abuse

▶ INFORMED CONSENT

Informed consent is the process by which patients knowingly and voluntarily agree to a treatment or procedure. In order to make informed decisions, patients must be given the following information:
- Name and purpose of treatment
- Potential risks and benefits
- Alternatives to the treatment
- Consequences of refusing treatment

In addition, opportunity must be given for the patient to ask questions, and he or she must have *capacity* to make an informed decision (see definition of capacity below).

Situations That Do Not Require Informed Consent

Informed consent need not be obtained in the following cases:
- Lifesaving medical emergency
- Suicide or homicide prevention (hospitalization)
- Minors—must obtain consent from parents *except* when giving obstetric care, treatment for sexually transmitted diseases (STDs), treatment for substance abuse (laws vary by state). In these cases, consent may be obtained from the minor directly, and information must be kept confidential from parents.

Emancipated Minors

Emancipated minors are considered competent to give consent for all medical care without input from their parents. Minors are considered emancipated if they:
- Are self-supporting
- Are in the military
- Are married
- Have children

▶ COMPETENCE VERSUS CAPACITY

Competence and *capacity* are terms that refer to a patient's ability to make informed treatment decisions. *Competence* is a legal term and can only be decided by a judge, whereas *capacity* is a clinical term and may be assessed by physicians.

Decisional capacity is *task specific* and can fluctuate over time; that is, a patient may have capacity to make one treatment decision while lacking capacity to make others. It is therefore important to assess capacity on a treatment-specific basis.

Assessment of Capacity

A patient is considered to have decisional capacity if he or she meets the following four criteria:

1. Can communicate a choice or preference
2. Understands the relevant information regarding treatment—purpose, risks, benefits, and alternatives; patient must be able to explain this information to you
3. Appreciates the situation and its potential impact or consequences according to his or her own value system and understands the ramifications of refusing treatment
4. Can logically manipulate information regarding the situation and reach rational conclusions

Criteria for determining capacity may be more stringent if the consequences of a patient's decision are very serious.

Assessing the Risk of Violence

The following factors increase the likelihood of a patient's becoming violent:
- History of violence
- Specific threat with a plan
- History of impulsivity
- Psychiatric diagnosis
- Substance abuse

The most important factor in assessing a patient's risk of violence is a history of violence.

▶ **COMPETENCE TO STAND TRAIL**

A fundamental tenet to the U.S. Criminal Code is that people who are mentally incompetent should not be tried. To stand trial, a person must:
- Understand the charges against him or her
- Have the ability to work with an attorney
- Understand possible consequences
- Be able to testify

▶ **NOT GUILTY BY REASON OF INSANITY**

In general, to be found *not guilty by reason of insanity*, one must have a mental illness, not understand right from wrong, and not understand consequences of actions *at the time the act was committed*. Depending on the state, one of the following **statutory criteria** must be met:

1. *M'Naghten:* This is the most stringent test and is standard in most jurisdictions. It assesses whether the person understands the nature, consequences, and wrongfulness of his or her actions.
2. *American Law Institute Model Penal Code: Cognitive prong* determines whether the person understands the wrongfulness of his or her actions, and *volitional prong* assesses whether he or she is able to act in accordance with the law.
3. *Durham:* This is the most lenient test and is rarely used; it assesses whether the person's criminal act has resulted from mental illness.

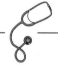

Insanity:
Criteria vary from state to state.

Crime requires "evil intent" (*mens rea*) and an "evil deed" (*actus reus*).

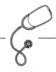

4 **D**s of malpractice: **D**ereliction (neglect) of a **D**uty that led **D**irectly to **D**amages

Malpractice is considered a tort or civil wrong rather than a crime. To successfully argue a case of malpractice against a physician, the patient must prove the following three conditions:

1. There is an established standard of care.
2. The physician breached his or her responsibility to the plaintiff.
3. The physician's breach of responsibility caused injury or damage to the plaintiff.

Compensatory damages are awarded to the patient as reimbursement for medical expenses, lost salary, or physical suffering. **Punitive damages** are awarded to the patient only in order to "punish" the doctor for gross negligence or carelessness.

Awards
and Opportunities
for Students Interested
in Psychiatry

American Academy of Child & Adolescent Psychiatry Medical Student Membership

AACAP membership for medical students costs $35/year and includes the following benefits:

- Subscriptions to the monthly Journal (both hard copy and online versions) ($124) and AACAP News ($70)
- Reduced fees for CME programs: a 6-day Annual Meeting, a 2-day January Psychopharmacology Update Institute, a 3-day Mid-Year Institute, and a 4-day Review Course for the Child Board Exams ($500)
- Five new Facts for Families, bringing the total to 78. Also available in Spanish to use in your practice ($35)
- Guidelines regarding the use of psychiatrists' signature ($10)
- Biographical Directory 2000 ($50), available for online search and update
- JobSource: List your vitae for free, place an ad ($50)
- National initiative to educate policy makers about the need to improve services for children and adolescents with mental illnesses and to ensure access of patients to child and adolescent psychiatrists
- Representation in the AMA House of Delegates
- AACAP home page—over 3 million hits per year
- Recruitment Kit and Code of Ethics
- 60 Committees, Task Forces, Managed Care Help Line, and CPT Code Module and Support Line

AMERICAN PSYCHIATRIC ASSOCIATION LISTSERV FOR MEDICAL STUDENTS

The APA Education Listserv is a bidirectional method of communication between the APA, medical students, residents, residency training directors, and others, to share information, comments, and suggestions of interest and concern to medical students and residents. To subscribe to this listserv, please visit APA's website at http://www.psych.org or e-mail your request to join to *ndelanoche@psych.org*. *Free registration for medical students at the Annual Meeting of the American Psychiatric Association.*

American Academy of Addiction Psychiatry Medical Student Memberships

The AAAP offers subsidized medical student memberships. Medical students are eligible for a 1-year membership in the American Academy of Addiction Psychiatry at the discounted rate of $45. Membership benefits include:

- Subscription to the quarterly, scholarly *The American Journal on Addictions*
- Subscription to *AAAP News*, the official quarterly newsletter of the Academy
- Opportunities to meet and network with experienced addiction clinicians, researchers, and faculty
- Discounts for meetings and products
- Access to Members-Only Area of AAAP Web site

Contact: American Academy of Addiction Psychiatry, 7301 Mission Road, Suite 252, Prairie Village, KS 66208; Fax: 913-262-4311

American Academy of Child & Adolescent Psychiatry

AACAP offers four awards for medical students:

1. $2,200 stipend for underrepresented minority students to work with a clinical psychiatrist mentor.

2. Jeanne Spurlock Research Summer Fellowship in drug abuse and addiction to work with a research psychiatrist mentor, for minority (including Asian) students. Five awards of $2,500 each are available. Awards also cover attendance at the Annual Meeting.

3. James Comer Minority Research Fellowship to work with a research psychiatrist mentor. This award provides five awards of $2,200 each plus 5 days at the AACAP Annual Meeting.

4. Jeanne Spurlock Minority Clinical Fellowship. This award provides five $2,500

fellowships for work during the summer with a child and adolescent psychiatrist mentor plus 5 days at the AACAP Annual Meeting.

For more information, contact: AACAP Office of Research and Training, 3615 Wisconsin Avenue NW, Washington, DC 20016; Phone: 202-966-7300; Fax: 202-966-2891

American Psychiatric Association PMRTP Summer Training Award for Underrepresented Minority Medical Students

The Program for Minority Research Training in Psychiatry (PMRTP) is a summer research fellowship funded by the National Institute of Mental Health and administered by the American Psychiatric Association (APA). The PMRTP is designed to increase the number of underrepresented minority men and women in the field of psychiatric research. Support is available for training opportunities during an elective period (3- to 6-month rotation) or as a summer experience. Funding for a summer training experience is available to minority medical students enrolled in accredited schools. Trainees must be U.S. citizens or permanent residents. Preference in selection goes to the underrepresented minorities given priority by the U.S. Department of Health and Human Services in awarding supplements in biomedical and behavioral research. These include American Indians, Blacks/African Americans, Hispanics, Pacific Islanders, or other ethnic or racial group members who have been found to be underrepresented in biomedical or behavioral research nationally.

Contact: Request selection criteria, an application, or other information by writing to Ernesto A. Guerra, Project Manager, or by calling 1-800-852-1390 or 202-682-6225; e-mail: eguerra@psych.org. You may also write to the Director of the PMRTP, James W. Thompson, MD, MPH.

AMERICAN SOCIETY OF CLINICAL HYPNOSIS AWARDS

Cash awards and recognition for the best papers written by a student on the subject of hypnosis. Papers may be clinical, theoretical, or the report of a research project. First prize will be $350, second prize $250, third prize $150. There will be five honorable mentions of $50 each. *Contact:* American Society of Clinical Hypnosis, 130 East Elm Court, Suite 201, Roselle, IL 60172-2000; Phone: 630-980-4740; Fax: 630-351-8490; E-mail: info@asch.net

Center for Chemical Dependency Treatment and Scaife Family Foundation Student Clerkship

Three-week clerkship involving both a clinical experience and a lecture series and providing information and experience, which will increase the awareness of the participants with respect to issues such as alcohol and other drug addiction, comorbidity and chemical dependency, and intervention methods for patients who abuse alcohol and other drugs. *Contact:* Dr. Janice Pringle, St. Francis Medical Center—Center for Chemical Dependency Treatment, 9th Floor, 400 45th Street, East Building, Pittsburgh, PA 15201; Phone: 412-622-8069

JOSEPH COLLINS FOUNDATION AWARD

An award based on both financial need and scholastic record and standing (upper half of class); a demonstrated interest in arts and letters or other cultural pursuits outside the field of medicine; indication of intention to consider specializing in neurology, psychiatry, or becoming a general practitioner; evidence of good moral character. Average grant is $2,500. *Contact:* Joseph Collins Foundation Attn: Secretary-Treasurer 153 East 53rd Street New York, NY 10022

Thomas Detre Prize

Sponsored by the University of Pittsburgh, Department of Psychiatry. The prize is for the best paper in any area of general psychiatry. $300 prize

Puig–Antich Memorial Prize

Sponsored by the University of Pittsburgh, Department of Psychiatry, this prize is for the best paper in any area of child or adolescent psychiatry. $300 prize

PRESIDENT'S COMMITTEE ON MENTAL RETARDATION SCHOLARSHIP

Scholarship offered to graduate students for advanced study in the field of mental retardation. Students must be able to document an economic need and a significant amount of volunteer

155

activity with mentally retarded persons. *Contact:* PCMR, 370 L'Enfant Promenade SW, Suite 701, Washington, DC 20447-0001; Phone: 202-619-0634; Fax: 202-205-9519

American Medical Association Rock Sleyster Memorial Scholarship

This fund provides scholarships to be awarded to U.S. citizens enrolled in accredited American or Canadian medical schools. Scholarships are given annually to assist needy and deserving students studying medicine who aspire to specialize in psychiatry. All nominees must be rising seniors. The award is $2,500. *Contact:* American Medical Association Education and Research Foundation, 515 North State Street, Chicago, IL 60610; Phone: 312-464-5357; Fax: 312-464-5973; *www.ama-assn.org*

American Academy of Addiction Psychiatry

The American Academy of Addiction Psychiatry is pleased to announce the annual Medical Student Award. This award provides a travel stipend for a medical student who is interested in the diagnosis, root causes, and treatment of addictive disorders. The award will be presented at the Annual Meeting and Symposium of the Academy. The recipient of the award will be invited to attend the AAAP Annual Meeting and Symposium to receive the award. Registration fees will be waived, and airfare and hotel costs will be paid for the Medical Student Award winner (up to $1,000). Interested students need to submit a curriculum vitae and a brief (less than 500 words) essay about their interest and achievements in the addictions to: American Academy of Addiction Psychiatry, 7301 Mission Road, Suite 252, Prairie Village, KS 66208; Fax: 913-262-4311

BETTY FORD SUMMER INSTITUTE FOR MEDICAL STUDENTS

The Summer Institute for Medical Students is a unique, quality learning experience for medical students wishing to gain greater understanding and insight into addictive disease and the recovery process. Mrs. Ford strongly shows her commitment to expanding the awareness of the health and human services professional community by endorsing this program and making it available to medical students across the country. *Contact:* Dr. James West, Betty Ford Center Training Department, 39000 Bob Hope Drive, Rancho Mirage, CA 92270; Phone: 760-773-4108; Toll free: 800-854-9211, Ext. 4108; Fax: 760-773-1508

AWARDS FOR MINORITY STUDENTS

Fellowship in Academic Medicine for Minority Students

Sponsored by the National Medical Fellowships, Inc., and underwritten by Bristol-Myers Squibb, each year up to 35 students are selected as Academic Medicine Fellows by the Program Development Committee and awarded grants of $6,000 each. The stipend enables each student to spend 8 to 12 weeks on a research project of interest under the guidance of an experienced biomedical researcher who acts as the student's mentor and who may use up to $2,000 of the fellowship grant to cover the costs of the internship. *Contact:* The Fellowship in Academic Medicine for Minority Students, National Medical Fellowships, Inc., 5 Hanover Square, 5th Floor, New York, NY 10004; Phone: 212-483-8880; *www.nmf-online.org*

National Medical Association Research Award

Symposium for minority residents and medical students to present original research and writing in the areas of clinical practice, neuropharmacology, psychophysiology, or behavioral medicine. Travel expenses available to selected participants. *Contact:* National Medical Association, 1012 Tenth Street NW, Washington, DC 20001; Phone: 202-347-1895; Fax: 202-842-3293

http://www.aaap.org/early/faq.html

This Web site, hosted by the American Academy of Addiction Psychiatry, is a resource for medical students, residents, and early-career psychiatrists. It has answers to frequently asked questions about a career in addiction psychiatry. This site also contains a mentor list of senior clinicians with their e-mail addresses, information on fellowship training, and other career info.

http://www.admsep.org/studentelectives.html

This link contains the Association of Directors of Medical Student Education in Psychiatry (ADMSEP) National Psychiatry Rotation Electives Catalogue. The purpose of these national opportunity listings are to assist senior medical students in finding and learning more about elective rotations offered at sites other than their parent institution.

http://www.vh.org/Providers /Lectures/EmergencyMed/ Psychiatry/TOC.html

This site, hosted by Virtual Hospital, contains the University of Iowa Hospitals and Clinics Emergency Psychiatry Service Handbook online.

http://www.aadprt.org/public/students.html

Hosted by the American Association of Directors of Psychiatric Residency Training (AADPRT), here medical students can find useful information and links on the Match, including a list of linked psychiatry training programs.

http://www.amsa.org/psych /mentors.cfm

Hosted by the American Medical Student Association, this site provides a list of psychiatry mentors for medical students.

http://members.aol.com/aglpnat/homepage.htm

The Association of Gay and Lesbian Psychiatrists (AGLP) is a professional organization of psychiatrists, psychiatry residents, and medical students that serves as a voice for the concerns of lesbians and gay men within the psychiatric community. The Association is committed to fostering a more accurate understanding of homosexuality, opposing discriminatory practices against gay men and lesbians, and promoting supportive, well-informed psychiatric care for lesbian and gay patients. The organization provides opportunities for affiliation and collaboration among psychiatrists who share these concerns.

Index

Awards/opportunities for students interested in psychiatry
(*continued*)
membership and subscriptions
(*continued*)
American Psychiatric Association Listserv For Medical Students, 154
minority students
Fellowship in Academic Medicine for Minority Students, 156
National Medical Association Research Award, 156
websites of interest
American Academy of Addiction Psychiatry, 157
American Association of Directors of Psychiatric Residency Training, 157
American Medical Student Association, 157
Association of Directors of Medical Student Education in Psychiatry, 157
Association of Gay and Lesbian Psychiatrists, 157
University of Iowa, 157
Virtual Hospital, 157

B

Barbiturates, 67
Bargaining stage of dying, elderly patients/residents and, 83
Behavior
children and disruptive, 91–92
dependent personality disorder, 57–58
histrionic personality disorder, 55, 58
mental status examination, 10
phobias, 42
Pick's disease, 78
repetitive/stereotyped, 86, 94
schizophrenia, 19, 20
schizotypal personality disorder, 52
See also Relationships; *individual disorders/diseases*
Behavioral therapy
agoraphobia, 41
anorexia nervosa, 116
autistic disorder, 94
binge-eating disorder, 117
borderline personality disorder, 54
conditioning, 135
enuresis, 97
generalized anxiety disorder, 46
learning theory, 134
major depressive disorder, 32
nicotine, 72
obsessive–compulsive disorder, 44

obsessive–compulsive personality disorder, 59
overview, 134
phobias, 42
pyromania, 112
schizophrenia, 22
sexual disorders, 127–128
techniques
aversion therapy, 135
biofeedback, 40, 109, 135
desensitization, systemic, 135
flooding and implosion, 135
token economy, 135
See also Aversive conditioning/therapy
Behavior on the wards, success in the psychiatry clerkship and
addressing patients/staff in a respectful way, 3
boundaries with patients, maintaining, 2
dressing in a professional manner, 2
exam, preparing for the, 4–5
hierarchy, awareness of the, 3
information, patient, 4
pleasant manner, acting in a, 3
respect for field of psychiatry/patients, 2
responsibility for patients, taking, 3
rights, respecting patients', 3
team player, being a, 4
volunteering, 4
Benadryl (diphenhydramine hydrochloride), 120, 143
Benign senescent forgetfulness, 83
Benzene and anxiety disorders, 38
Benzodiazepines
advantages of, 146
alcohol, 64, 146
Alzheimer's disease, 77
antipsychotics, 23
caffeine, 72
elderly patients/residents, 86
examples of, 146
gamma-aminobutyric acid, 146
generalized anxiety disorder, 46
panic disorder, 40
phencyclidine, 70
phobias, 42
vascular dementia, 77
Bereavement and elderly patients/residents, 85
Beta-adrenergic receptors, 30
Beta blockers
antipsychotics, 23
avoidant personality disorder, 57
phobias, 42
psychosis, 19
Betty Ford Summer Institute, 156

Binge-eating disorder
diagnosis and DSM-IV criteria, 117
overview, 117
treatment, 117–118
Biofeedback
defining terms, 135
pain disorders, 109
panic disorders, 40
Bipolar I disorder
course and prognosis, 33
diagnosis and DSM-IV criteria, 32
epidemiology, 33
etiology, 33
treatment, 33
Bipolar II disorder
course and prognosis, 34
diagnosis and DSM-IV criteria, 33
epidemiology, 33
etiology, 34
treatment, 34
Bladder control and childhood disintegrative disorder, 95
Blindness
conversion disorder, 106, 107
Creutzfeldt–Jakob disease, 80
Blood
antipsychotics, 23
carbamazepine, 145
dementia, 75
factitious disorder, 109
lithium, 145
valproic acid, 145
Blood alcohol level (BAL), 63
Blood pressure
antipsychotics, 23
cocaine, 65
delirium, 81
phencyclidine, 70
Body dysmorphic disorder
clinical vignette, 108
course and prognosis, 108
defining terms, 108
diagnosis and DSM-IV criteria, 108
epidemiology, 108
treatment, 108
Borderline mental retardation, 14
Borderline personality disorder (BPD)
course, 54
dependent personality disorder *vs.*, 58
diagnosis and DSM-IV criteria, 54
differential diagnosis, 54
epidemiology, 54
histrionic personality disorder *vs.*, 55
overview, 54
treatment, 54
trichotillomania, 114
Boundaries and family therapy, 136
Boundaries with patients and success in the psychiatry clerkship, maintaining, 2
Bovine spongiform encephalopathy, 80